A Way with Cancer:

A Cancer Cure Guide
for Serious
Do-It-Yourselfers

A Way with Cancer:

A Cancer Cure Guide
for Serious
Do-It-Yourselfers

Independent researchers have known for a long
time how to prevent, control and cure cancer;
however their results and practical know-how does
not reach the general public. This book will change
that. Learn how to prevent cancer and find how
others have fought it successfully.

Dick Schuyt, RPT

Second edition, 2015.

First print in 2003,
Then titled: Be Your Body's Cancer Coach.

Printed in the United States of America

Dedicated to two friends and heroes

Ans and Rinse Conradie

Perseverance under trial.

Exercising faith when challenged.

A fight well fought!

Table of Contents

Foreword

We write 2015. In the coming years one out of four Americans will be confronted with the dreaded diagnosis of...cancer. Almost 560,000 of them will die of this horrible disease in one year. In victim-numbers, it is the equivalent of a 9/11 calamity happening every other day of the year!

The costs for cancer are a whopping $156.7 billion per year ($ 156,700,000,000). Meanwhile, the costs for drugs are being increased every year by fifteen percent.

On top of that we have to add other facts, which make a realistic look into the future really grim. We still do not have a grip on air, soil and water pollution. Research tells us that we should not eat ocean fish, like salmon, any longer, since more and more heavy metals like mercury are found in the meat. Our vegetables have been found to decrease in nutritional value, and more vegetables and grains are being messed with genetically, predisposing us for a worldwide calamity.

Vitamins and minerals are being washed and bleached out of our daily foods by the food industries. Every year more hazardous carcinogens and toxic chemicals are being added to the stuff we put in our mouths, like toothpaste, diet sodas, drugs, hydrogenated oils, artificial sweeteners, etc.

The recent war activities in the Middle East have diseased many ex-combat personnel because of the use of depleted uranium. The fallout of this deadly stuff has reached the skies within our borders as well. Respiratory problems in America are on the rise, probably caused by radiation in the air we breathe.

To make our prospects look really ugly, we have to realize that the federal Food and Drug Administration (FDA), the American Medical Association (AMA) and the American Cancer Society have shown not to be interested at all in simple, *unpatented* treatments for cancer that have healed people as far back as before the Second World War. They even take an aggressive stand against anyone who dares to claim that there is a cure for cancer. Even writing about cures can make you end up in jail.

Yep, it is an ugly picture of the years to come.

What does this mean for you? It means that you will seriously have to start thinking about three questions:

- how can I prevent my body from getting cancer?

- how can I test my body to see if it is a possible candidate for cancer?

- how can I successfully help my body to get rid of cancer after I have been diagnosed with it?

The answers to all of these questions you will find in the following chapters.

Preface

This is a book filled with hope. Not the kind of hope that lies far away in the distant future, unreachable for most people, but real, short-term, honest-to-goodness hope that can be realized in days, weeks and in severe cases several months. You'll learn how to prevent cancer. Period!

If you have been labeled with the seemingly hopeless diagnosis of cancer or if cancer runs in your family and you live in constant fear, this book will be a blessing to you. First of all, you will learn how to do a simple test that will tell you the state of health of your tissues and of the fluid that floats around the cells. The result of this test can tell you if your body is susceptible to cancer and other diseases, or not. Yes, there really is such a test and yes, you can do it by yourself, at home.

If you have been diagnosed with cancer, the following chapters will tell you much about how to take back control and how to help your body heal itself. You will read about scientists who have found ways to get rid of cancer. You will read how you can apply their discoveries to coach your body back to wellness. You will also read about terminally ill people who found their health again.

This book is filled with so much hope, that after you have read it, your head will spin. You will put it down and say to yourself, "This is too good to be true. It's just unbelievable. Why haven't I heard about this before?" (These questions will be answered as well.)

Probably after a good night's sleep, you will pick it up again in the morning and you will say to yourself, *"OK, I'm ready, I'm going to lick this thing! I'm back in the race and I'll take the driver's seat!"*

> Take courage!
>
> Professionals built the Titanic
>
> ...but it was an amateur like you
>
> who built the ark!

Introduction

---

*In a time of universal deceit, telling the
truth is a revolutionary act.*
- George Orwell

Twelve years ago I immigrated with my wife and four children from the Netherlands in Europe to the beautiful state of Florida, where I now work as a physical therapist, visiting people in their homes. It is my job to assist in physical rehabilitation after someone has gone through surgery or other treatment in the hospital. I love my job. It's personal. It's hands-on. I can make a difference in someone's life.

Every so often I visit cancer patients who are undergoing the usual treatment of chemotherapy, radiation and/or surgery. As the weeks progress I often see them decline in function until some become bed-ridden, often living in agony. This week, as I write this, I visited a fifty-year-old cancer patient with a tumor in the brain that, every year, keeps coming back.

Let's call her Esther. Esther is a single grandma, taking care of a ten-year-old grandson. Every year she goes through chemotherapy. Every year another chunk of her body is destroyed by cancer, but also by the side effects of the chemotherapy.

Now the cancer has come back again. The left side of her body is paralyzed. Esther cannot stand by herself anymore and has difficulty walking; that is why she needs physical therapy. She is without vision in one eye. The feeling in her left arm is completely gone. While her mother helps her walk, Esther tends to bump into doorposts, walls and furniture. Her balance is compromised. Often she does not make it to the bathroom in time.

Esther is "lucky"; she still has both of her parents who are willing to take care of her and her grandson. Her doctor, I'm sure, has told her many times that the treatment she is receiving is the best that science can offer her. "There is nothing more we can do for you..." Esther's church community is praying for her. But time is ticking away...

I have many of these stories to tell. Joe is a sixty-year-old man who, after chemo treatment and radiation, could not get up from his bed anymore. He was scared to get up. Everything would start to turn in his head when he tried to walk.

Or Ethel, sixty-three, who did well after the first three treatments and then after the fourth one lost all her strength and will to live.

The doctors told them all: "It is the best we can do for you..." I have come to the point where I cannot stand it any more. I am in a slow burn. All these patients I told you about–but you too–were told a lie. A blatant lie. The truth is that people have been and are being cured from cancer *right now*. Books have been and are written about successful treatments of cancer. Doctors go on record stating that it is "easy to cure cancer."

The Internet is buzzing with websites trying to get the truth out to those who have fallen ill or to anyone who has an interest in this. There is a lot of truth out there, but it does not reach those people who need to hear it: the cancer patients. Your doctor does not have the time to read it, simply because he tries to keep up with the magazines from the pharmaceutical industry.

The media are biased, as we all know, and lean towards the industries with the deep pockets.

The FDA, your medical watchdog agency, and even the AMA (the American Medical Association) will sue every doctor who steps out of line and will see to it that proven alternatives for drugs cannot be sold in this once-free country. The truth is being pushed under and the good news does not reach the general public. They are the ones who need it most and who are scared out of their wits after hearing that they have the "dreaded disease."

Let's go back to Esther. She had had cancer for five years already. She'd had multiple surgeries and radiation treatments, and several drugs had been tried out on her, but no medical professional had ever talked with her about the many and very successful alternative cancer treatments. I find that offensive. It is inhumane and un-American.

Something needs to change. That is what this book is about: an attempt to make you aware of the dangers of the accepted treatments and to inform you about the good news–there are ways to control cancer! Cancer is not a death sentence. There is life after cancer and you can live happily ever after.

This little book is for those people who probably will never read a medical book or who do not have access to the information highway, the Internet. Written in short sleeve, kitchen table English, with a minimum of technical details, and no footnotes referring to unreadable research papers.

When you read on, do not forget that I am not a doctor! I am a physical therapist and as such I am not trained, nor licensed to make any medical diagnosis or give advice, nor am I trained in the knowledge of medications.

Forget even that I am a physical therapist. I am just a bystander like you, looking at an epidemic taking place and trying to lend a helping hand to my family and to the people I meet every day.

Cancer has grabbed my interest since I've seen what this awful disease has done to some dear people. Consequently I started reading about the research that has been and is being done. The more I read the more frustrated I became, until I could not stand it anymore and started to list many very promising ways to control cancer. The result is in the pages you are reading.

Before we get into the details of how to kick cancer in the rear end, there is something that begs for an explanation. You will still have this thought in the back of your mind that keeps nagging you: "if there is so much truth out there about successful cancer treatments, why doesn't my doctor know it and inform me about this. Why do I not hear or see anything about it in the media?" Before we go into the good stuff I need to explain to you why your doctor behaves the way he does.

In shorthand. In the early nineteen hundreds the medical universities in America were in very poor shape financially. Many were on the brink of closing their doors, mainly because of a lack of funds. However, grant money from the Rockefeller and Carnegie foundations reached and saved many of these universities. Along with the money that poured in, came powerful men, connected to these foundations, who took places in the boards of directors of these universities to make sure that the interests of the foundations were being served accordingly.

The foundations were tax-exempt havens for the extremely rich and powerful, especially for those who made zillions of dollars in the oil and pharmaceutical industries. These pharmaceutical, tax-exempt foundations influenced the university boards in how to write the curricula. (This is all a matter of historical, public record that anyone can read in old newspapers and books in the library.) The training for doctors started leaning heavily towards the use of chemicals we call medications and the use of diagnostic equipment. I hope you now understand why, after almost every doctor's visit, you come home with another prescription for a new medicine.

The pharmaceutical industries tell the universities what to teach the medical students, but also what *not* to teach. That is why your doctor, of all healthcare professionals, knows little about diet. He has hardly learned anything about the importance of foods, nutrition, vitamins, herbs, minerals, supplements, because all of these things are not profitable to the pharmaceutical business owners.

Let's never forget this: **pharmaceutical companies** (pharmacomps) are *businesses*. Their directors have to answer to shareholders who are not happy when there is no profit being made. The way to generate more profit is to sell more drugs to more people. People will only buy drugs if they need them or if they think they need them. The need for drugs is driven by disease and so we can conclude that:

> for drug companies *disease is profit.*
>
> The ongoing *treatment* of disease is the continuation of *profit*.
>
> The increase of disease means an increase of treatment, which is the increase of profit.

Here is another thing that we have to keep in mind: drugs are special products. They are like books. They all have a copyright or a "patent" so that only the "inventor" of a particular drug may produce and sell it.

For example, the drug "aspirin" was developed by the Bayer Company. Bayer went to the patent office and received a patent for this 'man made' chemical substance that we now call aspirin. Nobody else was allowed to produce, market and sell aspirin without Bayer's approval. This of course put the Bayer Company in a very fortunate position. They and only they can set the sales price for aspirin. There is no competition with other companies about this product and that allows Bayer to make as much profit with aspirin as they want. Isn't that a nice business?

Maybe you will say now, "Well, what's wrong about an industry making a profit?"

Let's go a bit deeper into the rabbit hole.

Have you ever wondered why you hardly see any commercials on TV about vitamins, like vitamin C?

Vitamin C is a wonderful substance that keeps us from contracting many different diseases. Many studies have found it to be very beneficial for our health and even curative for many different diseases.

Well, the answer is: a vitamin is a natural substance that cannot be patented. Anyone can produce and sell it resulting in price competition and subsequently a low profit margin. I can buy a pound of vitamin C in my vitamin shop for less than $15. Try that with aspirin!

The pharmacomps are not interested in products they cannot patent, even if these products would be highly beneficial and curative, for two reasons. First of all the product cannot be sold with the desired profit and secondly the curative aspect of the product would be counter productive to the business.

You ask why? Well, the increased use of vitamin C would help the general population to become healthier. In many cases it would even eliminate their state of disease, which in turn would generate less income to the drug business, because a patient cured is ...a customer lost.

It goes even deeper. Besides their disinterest with vitamins the pharmacomps have shown on occasions in the past to be unwilling to develop drugs that would mean a downright cure for a disease.

In the case of cancer for instance, it was Dr. Wilburn Ferguson who, during his stay with the Amazon Indians, had discovered a natural potion that cured most of his cancer patients. When he asked one of the pharma giants that researched his potion why they did not follow up on their positive findings, he was simply told that they acknowledged the effectiveness of his potion but that they were not interested, because mass production would destroy their business.

More recent is the research on leaves from the Graviola tree. The working ingredient "annonacin", found in these leaves, has been researched and proven to kill certain cancers. For years scientists from certain pharmacomps have been trying in their laboratories to alter the annonacin just slightly without losing its effectiveness in fighting cancer. All for the obvious reason: the natural substance annonacin put on the free market would hardly generate a profit, but a slightly-altered chemical annonacin would allow the pharmacomp to file for a patent after which they would control the price of the "newly found" cancer drug and make another fortune.

So can end a perfectly natural and cheap cure for cancer into a chemically-altered, needlessly expensive drug, probably with all sorts of side effects for which of course you will need additional drug treatment.

In the case of Graviola, a pharmacomp tried for years to alter annonacin into a drug but did not succeed. So when they could not patent the annonacin they simply pulled the plug on the research and walked away, leaving millions of people without hope. (Read more on how to use Graviola in Chapter 9.)

To give you an idea of the kind of profits that the pharmacomps are making, you may want to read the following. In an article called, *"The shocking truth behind prescription drug prices,"* William Faloon in "Life Extension Magazine" compared the price of several drugs with the cost-price of the generic active ingredient in the drug, that is often manufactured outside the USA. The popular stomach acid suppressing drug Prilosec, for example, sells for $360.00 per one hundred capsules.

> The total cost of the active ingredient for one hundred capsules of Prilosec is only ...fifty-two cents!!
>
> **This makes a nice profit of 69,417%.**
>
> Yes, a whopping sixty nine thousand four hundred and seventeen percent profit!

I hear you sigh by now: "Is anybody looking out for me?"

Well, as we've seen, the drug industry isn't ...really. And, being a business, they are not really obliged to us to come up with a cure for cancer and shoot themselves in the foot at the same time. They are in the market for a profit and, irony of ironies, many of us share the financial benefit of their success, since the money of our 401Ks and pension funds is being invested through the stock market in their companies. Almost literally we are building our financial fortune over our own over-medicated bodies.

So, then who is looking out for me? The FDA (Food and Drug Administration), the federal medical watchdog? Surely my government will look after me and protect me from harm, won't it?

The following statement was made by Dr. David Graham, senior drug safety researcher with the FDA, when he was interviewed in 2004 by Manette Loudon:

Since November, when I appeared before the Senate Finance Committee and announced to the world that the FDA was incapable of protecting America from unsafe drugs or from another Vioxx, very little has changed on the surface and substantively nothing has changed. The structural problems that exist within the FDA, where the people who approve the drugs are also the ones who oversee the post marketing regulation of the drug, remain unchanged. The people who approve a drug when they see that there is a safety problem with it are very reluctant to do anything about it because it will reflect badly on them. They continue to let the damage occur. America is just as at risk now, as it was in November, as it was two years ago, and as it was five years ago.

To show you how the interests of the food and drug industry are being intertwined with our governmental agencies: recently the former FDA commissioner Lester M. Crawford resigned and joined a lobbying firm specializing in food and drug related issues. After a waiting period of one year he can lobby his former FDA colleagues and is allowed to offer advice to anyone about the FDA.

What about the AMA, the American Medical Association? Their staff must be taking my well being to heart.

Well, let's see, recently three medical doctors authored a paper to document the fact that nearly one million Americans are killed by modern medicine each year. This means that hospitals, pharmaceuticals and doctors are the number one cause of death in the United States. ("Death by Medicine," 2003, Carolyn Dean MD, Martin Feldman MD, Debora Rasio MD, Dorothy Smith PhD, Gary Null PhD).

Well then surely the American Cancer Societies will be on my side of the equation, won't they?

> "Everyone should know that most cancer research is largely a fraud and that the major cancer research organizations are derelict in their duties to the people who support them." - Linus Pauling PhD *(Two-time Nobel Prize winner)*

If we follow the money trail we will eventually come to the realization that all these spheres of interest run on money, and lots of it. Volumes can be filled describing the occasions where things pertaining to your and my well-being and interest were simply dumped into the waste basket.

OK, so my family doctor, my MD, he is in the business of looking out for me and my health, right?

Well, yes and no. Your doc may be a good and honest guy. A real people person. A guy who started his career with great intentions of helping his suffering fellow men and women. There must be many such doctors out there and if you have found one, stick to him or her.

Doctors live under enormous pressures nowadays. Have a look around in his or her office and you will find out. Nurses, administrative staff, maintenance people, expensive diagnostic equipment and paperwork! Doctors have become managers of *disease care centers.* They pay astronomical premiums to insurance companies to stay away from the many lawsuits that hang over their heads every day of the week.

They have to keep up with the demands of the drug culture that pulls from both sides. The pharmacomps keep inventing new diseases and cranking out new drugs with dozens of side effects that your doctor has to understand before he prescribes them to you. You and too many other patients are daily demanding his attention, having been "educated" in TV commercials and magazines about new drugs. You know them by heart: "Ask your doctor if Nexium is right for you!"

We cannot really expect a human being to juggle all these responsibilities and at the same time to have an open mind to all the details of *your* particular medical problem.

But let's say that you found the doctor who miraculously can do all that and more. In our United States of America doctors have to conform to the practice of "consensus medicine." If your cancer doctor advises you to do any other therapy than chemotherapy, radiation, or surgery, he takes a big chance of being labeled a "quack" by his medical peers, which can ultimately result in his license being revoked.

The AMA does not allow its members to step out of line. Without a license you cannot practice. Without a practice you cannot pay the bills. Now you know why your doctor tells you: "There is nothing more we can do for you."

The following chapters all have one thing in common: they all describe ways to assist your body in the healing process. Nobody can heal; not even the best trained doctor. God has created the body with innate healing intelligence. In Genesis we read that "God saw all that He had made, and behold, it was very good."

Healing happens because our beautiful, biological system is perfectly geared for survival. If only we give it what it needs and withhold from it what it cannot use, we will stay in good health until we simply die of "old age." This principle, however, is contrary to the conventional cancer treatments of chemo treatment (poisoning), surgery (cutting) and radiation (burning).

These therapies are not designed to help the body cure itself. They are designed to destroy only the tumor, but in the process they also destroy parts of our healthy tissue and they severely weaken our immune systems.

What your doctor may not tell you about cancer **surgery** is this:

"An objective appraisal is that the statistical rate of long term survival after surgery is, on the average at best, only ten or fifteen percent.

And once the cancer has metastasized to a second location, surgery has almost no survival value. The reason is that, like the other therapies approved by orthodox medicine, surgery removes only the tumor. It does not remove the cause" ("World without Cancer," pp. 141-142).

What you need to know about **radiation** is this: "X-ray therapy (radiation) is cursed with the same drawbacks of surgery. But it has one more: it actually increases the likelihood that cancer will develop in other parts of the body! Excessive exposure to radioactivity is an effective way to induce (cause) cancer" ("World without Cancer," p. 142).

And will your doc tell you the following about **chemo-therapy?** Read it and shiver.

"Poisoning the system is the objective of these drugs, and the resulting pain and illness often is a torment worse than the disease itself . The toxins catch the blood cells in the act of dividing and cause blood poisoning. The gastrointestinal system is thrown into convulsion causing nausea, diarrhea, loss of appetite, cramps and progressive weakness. Hair cells are fast growing, so the hairs fall out during treatment. Reproductive organs are affected causing sterility. The brain becomes fatigued. Eyesight and hearing are impaired. Every conceivable function is disrupted with such agony for the patient that many of them elect to die of the cancer rather than to continue the treatment."

And, says Dr. Ralph Moss, former Assistant Director of Public Relations at leading American cancer research facility Memorial Sloan Kettering, NY:

"In the end there is no proof that chemotherapy in the vast majority of cases actually extends life. This is the great lie about chemotherapy, that somehow there is a correlation between shrinking a tumor and extending the life of a patient."

These orthodox treatments are all geared towards taking away the "product" of cancer, which is: the tumor. However once the tumor is cut, poisoned or burned away, the cancer process can still be very much alive, wreaking havoc, especially since the cancer-cells have mutated because of the radiation and chemo-treatment, and have become super-resistant to future therapies. With a severely-pummeled immune system your body will hardly be able to stop a newly growing tumor. The treatments will, with the tumor, often destroy parts of your God-given body. It is like playing "Russian roulette" with a pistol loaded not with just one bullet, but with three.

Remember Esther? There was no cure. There was only treatment, and more treatment, and another treatment. And then there were bills and more bills.

There must be a better way. And there is!

But let's first have a look at cancer. Let's meet our enemy and see what he is like.

Introduction

I really hope that when you turn this page and start with the first chapter, you will not feel intimidated by this much feared word: *"cancer."* As you will find out, cancer is not a micro monster that is untamable and unstoppable, going on a rampage inside your body like an alien invader.

Where I grew up people only dared to mention the word *"cancer"* with a dimmed voice as if "it" could jump them at any time and any place. Nonsense, of course!

When you turn to the next chapter you will be the next person who has decided to look cancer in the face and who is not afraid to fight it head-on. It is time we shake off that uneasiness. It's time you start to intimidate cancer and kick some tumor-butt!

Chapter 1

What is Cancer?

Cancer (or neo-plasma) is the development of fast growing, placenta-like, cells. Let's call these cells super-growers, or SGs. When these SGs are situated in the ovary of a woman, they will grow and multiply rapidly after conception into a placenta and an umbilical cord to function in the nourishing of the new embryo. Some of these same SGs can be found however in other places of the body, where they have a function in the repair of damaged tissue.

When a tornado hits your town and damages your house by blowing out a window you will quickly get some sheets of plywood to close up the hole.

So it is with the body. Damage can take place at any time and in many places of the body. This damage can be caused by cigarette smoke, toxins, radiation, chemicals, etc. The blood will immediately order the super-growers to the places of damage, where they will multiply quickly and differentiate into new tissue cells to replace the damaged ones. If they are not restrained by the normal hormonal processes, they will continue to grow uninhibited and randomly.

We could say that "over-healing" then takes place. A cluster of these cells grows into a …tumor. This is the process we call cancer.

Cancer happens when a perfectly normal and beneficial process is not stopped at the time that the repair is finished. The repair process is switched on, but not turned off at the right time. Only in this circumstance can uninhibited cell growth develop into a tumor.

Now you'll understand why we think that there are so many different things that can cause cancer. These things merely start the normal repair process. That is really all they do. And in a healthy situation the repair will run its normal course, bringing healing to a tissue and then simply cease.

Tumor growth is caused by the failure to inhibit and stop the repair process.

We will not go into all the details, but it is of interest to know that one of the restrainers that is missing in a group of cancerous tumor cells, is a certain vitamin, which will be discussed in Chapter 8.

Normal cells die after a certain life span; they self-destruct. This pre-programmed cell death called *apoptosis* does not take place in cancerous cells. They just keep on growing.

You will find that some of the natural anti-cancer substances that we'll talk about eliminate cancer because of their ability to restore normal cell death to the cancer cell. For now it is enough to know that cancer is an over-reaction of an otherwise normal function of our body, geared towards the repair of damaged tissue. This tissue-damage takes place in a number of different ways, every day and every minute. For instance, through radiation, by too much radiation from the sun, X-rays or nuclear waste, or through toxins or free-radicals.

> The real enemy then is the condition where our body somehow has become deficient in the necessary cancer-inhibitors so that an otherwise normal repair process runs amuck and causes a piling up of cells which we call a tumor.

Here is another thing that you need to know about cancer. Cells need and use oxygen to produce energy. A continual flow of oxygen-rich blood reaches the cells through the circulation.

Cancer cells somehow change over to a different kind of fuel: sugars! The question is whether they do this because of a lack of oxygen in their environment or because they have changed their programming somehow to burning sugars instead of oxygen.

Such change in program could have happened by a gene mutation, which you can compare to a "computer crash" in the nucleus of the cell which is the command center, or it could happen when the cell wall is damaged.

Cancer cells differ from normal (repair-) cells by four things:

- they do not differentiate into functional tissue cells,
- their growth is not inhibited,
- they use sugars for fuel in stead of oxygen,
- and they do not die at the normal time.

Growing a tumor is an extremely complex process. It takes a great variety of factors to ultimately lead to the growth of a tumor.

If you have ever ventured into the noble art of baking bread you'll have some understanding of how many things have to come together just right to get the right result.

Chapter 2

Baking a Loaf of Bread

I know this sounds preposterous but the growth of a cancerous tumor in your body is much like making a loaf of bread. Let me explain.

The process of making a nice loaf of bread is subject to several requirements. Certain conditions have to be met and ingredients have to be mixed together before you can start up the oven. The flour has to be of a certain consistency; the temperature of the water needs to be just right; salt should be added at the last possible moment so it will not interfere too much with the growing of the yeast in the dough; the yeast has to be fresh, etc, etc. Dozens of things have to come together just right to have a ball of sticky dough grow into a beautiful bread.

The baker has some knowledge of the processes that are going on inside the dough, however he is unaware of all the complicated changes in chemistry that take place and he does not fully understand all the reactions and dynamics that make the blob of dough into a loaf of bread. He just adds the ingredients, meets all the conditions and, *voila* (that's French), the dough will rise and the baker will have his bread.

Our physical body is a gift from God, who was very pleased with what He had made. He made our biological systems very well, geared for surviving the toughest challenges.

It is not easy to contract cancer. We do not grow a tumor simply because we didn't get enough sleep last night, or because we ate too much pizza.

For bread dough to rise or for cancer to become manifest, a lot of different factors need to happen and many conditions have to be met. A lung tissue cell can become cancerous, but before this cell can grow into a tumor an awful lot of ingredients have to be added at exactly the right time, in exactly the right amount and under exactly the right conditions.

For example; cancer cells can only grow and develop in an environment that is acidic. Alkalinity (the opposite of acid) kills the tumor process. So, one important condition in the development of a tumor is: the cell needs to be in an acidic environment.

Another requirement, as we've seen already, is a shortage of oxygen. Cancer does not survive in an environment that is rich in oxygen. So here we have already two conditions that are vital for tumor growth: acidity and a lack of oxygen.

By now you'll understand that if we will find the requirements, or contributing factors for developing a cancerous tumor, we can simply stop cancer from happening by turning the process around and take some, or better, all of these factors away! Right?

We do not have to be a doctor in oncology (a cancer doctor) to prevent or stop cancer from happening. We do not need to know exactly what cancer is or how, chemically, a tumor forms.

> If we know how to inhibit the cancer process, we can simply tune our bodies in such a way that cancer cannot grow or survive there.

Well, if that is the case, wouldn't you really like to know more about these ingredients that are so essential to the tumor growing process? Here are some of the things that science so far has come up with:

- Cancer is always seen together with a parasite named Fasciolopsis buskii, an intestinal fluke. (Yes, you may forget his name.)

- Cancer can only exist in an acidic environment; it cannot survive in an alkaline habitat.

- Cancer only happens in cells that have broken down and degenerated cell walls.

- Cancer feeds on sugar, not on oxygen like normal cells do. It cannot survive in an abundance of oxygen.

- Cancer cells can only develop in the absence of vitamin B_{17}, trypsin and progesterone.

- Cancer has a much better chance of developing when your immune system is weakened.

- Cancer is often ignited by severe and sudden mental trauma.

So now we've found seven important cancer ingredients, or factors. If you have been diagnosed with cancer, all these above named factors will be present in your body to some degree. You are growing a tumor just like a blob of dough that rises in the pan to become a loaf of bread.

This may be an overwhelming reality to you, seeing so many different factors contributing to growing a tumor in your body. You need some good news!

Here are some good tidings:

You do not need to eliminate *all* ingredients to stop your cancer. Doctors have cured people from cancer by just changing the environment of their cells from acidic to alkaline; or *just* by mending their broken down cell walls, or *just* by adding oxygen to the tumor.

There is ample "anecdotal evidence" in history to prove that cancer can be controlled and stopped by eliminating just a few of the necessary ingredients for cancer. Isn't that the best news you've read since your last cup of coffee?

But hang on; let's step back for a moment. When you have cancer, you will need to weigh all your options carefully.

There still are other options: surgery, chemo treatment, radiation. How do they relate to the "bread baking" situation?

You can still have the surgeon cut your tumor out, which will temporarily save you, but a surgery does not change anything about the ingredients. They will still be there, even after the surgery is over. The ingredients have set you up in a situation where you are predisposed for contracting cancer. As long as this predisposition is not eliminated, cancer can flare up again at any time just like a gasoline fire where the flames have been extinguished but a tiny spark can turn the place blazing again. A new cancerous tumor-process can start at anytime anywhere in your body since the tumor ingredients are still there!

Chemo treatment and radiation will not take away the ingredients either. Treatment can poison or burn away a tumor, but this too will leave the ingredients untouched. As a matter of fact, it even adds to the problem by ruining parts of your immune system, acidifying your tissues even further and dampening your spirit.

Maybe you have already gone through these treatments and you may have found that the cancer has come back again. Maybe you are going through chemo treatment right now. Or perhaps it is your first time and you have to decide what option is best for you.

Wherever you are in this process, whatever you decide and whatever route you take, somewhere down the line you will have to rid your body of the cancer ingredients. Only when you've eliminated the cancer ingredients, tumors will not grow back again.

So, what then can we do to eliminate each of the above mentioned ingredients, factors or requirements for cancer? That is what I'd like to talk to you about in the next chapters. It is not very difficult as you will see. Let's go through our list of seven again and look at each of them individually:

- We'll need to kill the parasite.

- We'll have to change our acidic cell environment to being alkaline again.

- We need to stop the degeneration of our cell walls and repair the damage.

- We'll need to increase the concentration of oxygen in the body

- Supplement with vitamin B_{17}, trypsin and progesterone.

- Our immune system needs a thorough overhaul.

- And last but not least; let's get rid of the wrong mindset and neutralize any cancer trigger asap.

The next chapters will give you practical advice on how to eliminate the ingredients of cancer. We will spend a chapter on every single factor and show you how you can steer your body back to normal.

In the literature on the history of cancer cures you can find many instances where cancer went into remission (this means the tumor growing process stopped) after the removal of only one ingredient.

So, let's make life miserable or rather impossible for your tumor and your cancer and take away *all seven of them!*

Or, do you still believe that there is nothing you can do against your cancer, since even the medical professionals have not found a cure for cancer? We need to talk some more...

Chapter 3

Getting the Right Perspective

We hardly hear anymore of the old disease known as scurvy, but between the sixteenth and the eighteenth centuries many a seaman died a horrible death due to the symptoms of this wretched sickness.

Naval fleets would sail the vast oceans on trips that took many months, returning with only a handful of men that had managed to stay alive. And so it went for centuries. Scurvy was identified by the symptoms, but nobody knew the cause of or the cure for it.

In 1747 James Lind, a surgeon's mate at the H.M.S. Salisbury, finally discovered that scurvy could be prevented and even cured with oranges and lemons. (Now we know that it is the vitamin C in the citrus fruit that prevents and cures scurvy.) So, although the exact *cause* of scurvy was still unknown, Lind had found a simple way to prevent and even cure this horrible, body-destroying disease that made thousands of casualties!

We would expect that from this moment on the problem of scurvy on board the ships would be eradicated. But no; the naval bureaucracy of Lind's day did not accept such a simple solution to their problem. It took more than forty years, and approximately more than 100,000 casualties, before the British Admiralty wrote an official order that one ounce of lemon juice per day was to be given to every sailor. Another agency, the British Board of Trade, took 112 years to adopt similar precautions.

In his book *The Healing Factor*, Irwing Stone mentions the ridiculous situation of sailors on board of merchant vessels, dying from scurvy, while delivering lemons to the ships of the Royal Navy!

While we're at it, during the American Civil War 30,000 cases of scurvy were reported, but it took the U.S. Army until 1895 to order lemons and oranges for their men.

A history of stubborn pride, closed minds and just plain carelessness. People were dying from scurvy by the thousands, but the medical bureaucracy looked in only one direction to find a cure that would bring healing and prestige. They turned a deaf ear to the ones who had found it already, sending their own sailors and soldiers to an early grave.

Doctor Semmelweis found the simple answer to infections that were killing so many women in the hospitals after childbirth: hand washing! It took a long before his peers took his advice seriously. And there are many more examples in history where doctors and healers found a downright cure before science ever laid hold of an explanation why. Antibiotics were used successfully against bacteria long before scientists deciphered the DNA code.

Now, before we dismiss these stories as freaks of history, let's read on and learn a little history about cancer treatments.

In 1924, more than eighty years ago, Otto Warburg won the Nobel Prize for discovering that cancer was associated with a lack of oxygen. In animals he could "switch" tumor growth on by lowering the oxygen content of their environment and "switch" it off by releasing the oxygen back in.

In the fifties Dr. Carl J. Reich found that many of his cancer patients became better after having them supplement with calcium, which neutralizes the acid in and around the cell.

Dr. K. Brewer and Dr. H. Sartori later found that cancer cells died when the acid overload in the cells was *completely* neutralized by treating their patients with Cesium and Rubidium, showing remarkable survival rates in a patient group that had already been given up by the doctors.

Of course we would expect the cancer institutes to pour large sums of money into new research that would follow up on these successes, to eradicate this dreadful disease once and for all.

A new age could have been heralded in, promising the victory over cancer. Well, you know the truth is quite the contrary. The quest and research for a bona fide cancer cure has since been driven underground. A continual struggle is going on in the world of cancer research between benevolence and profit, goodwill and money; up till now money and profit have always had the upper hand.

As with vitamin C and scurvy, the medical (read: pharmaceutical) bureaucracy is far, far behind on the facts, only looking in the direction of the development of patented drugs that bring a huge profit.

They are still looking at the extreme details, while others have already found ways to control and stop cancer. It will probably take many more decennia before the cures for cancers that have been found will be used in regular cancer treatment protocols.

> What we can learn from history is that we do not need to know the exact cause, origin or dynamics of a disease (cancer), to be able to prevent and eliminate it.

In the next chapters you will find a smorgasbord of all sorts of different approaches that inhibit your cancer and that can bring it to a grinding halt; all of them having a proven and documented track record in effectively pushing back cancer. All these approaches were pioneered by people who deserve a Nobel prize for their relentless pursuit of health, and their unfaltering search for ways to overcome disease. Their ultimate goal in life was and is to stop disease and human suffering.

We owe these men and women to be written in our halls of fame, however most of them have been and are now being persecuted by the medical and pharmaceutical establishment to the extent that most of us would give up. This is the reason why you have probably never heard of them.

They found a cure, or a control for a disease, which in itself is a threat to the multi-billion dollar medical "industry". Anyone who dares to come up with a cure for cancer finds himself in direct opposition to the enormously powerful pharmaceutical industry, which will not delay in defending its ultimate source of unbelievable high and continuing profits: *the continuation of disease.*

Many have found healing of their bodies from cancer by following the instructions of these pioneers of health. Their research and know-how has saved the lives of many people who were written off by the medical system.

Some of these pioneers that you will meet in the following chapters are medical doctors, some are not. They have, however, degrees in different sciences and their work has been accredited by medical doctors, who apply their discoveries in their own medical practices.

When we turn to them now to see how we can benefit from their hard work, we do it with gratitude, knowing that the fruit of their labor will lead us closer to the truth and nearer to becoming well again.

The following chapters will educate you in different ways to control cancer. Step by step you will find how you can help your body to get rid of the ingredients, or **factors** for cancer.

Each individual step has been proven and documented to inhibit and/or stop degenerative diseases like cancer, lupus, arthritis, and others. So why not do them all and make sure you do everything possible to get back on the road to wellness. You are on a destroyer mission!

Some steps will have almost immediate results, others may take weeks to fulfill. They are not arranged in sequential order, however you really want to start with step one, since it can keep your cancer at bay, while you are working hard on fulfilling the other steps. Most steps you need to do every day.

While you're at it, I advise you to stay connected to your physician. However, now that you are more informed about the severe side effects of the orthodox cancer "treatments," you may not want to jump head over heels into, for example, surgery. Now that you're on your way back to health, you may want to hold on to your gall bladder, your hair, your ovaries, or your breasts a little longer. You really look better with them!

All suggested recommendations for foods, vitamins, minerals and supplements, from here on, are for adult bodies.

In Appendix D you'll find a list of books that are recommended for those who want to dig a little deeper.

So, have a pleasant journey through the next chapters and, if you have been diagnosed with cancer, don't forget General Patton's definition of success:

It's
how high
you bounce back after
you've hit
rock

bottom.

Chapter 4

The Parasite Factor

*"Cancer is no longer the deadly disease
it once was. In fact you can clear it up in
less time than it takes to get a doctor's
appointment for a check up."*
-- Hulda Clark Ph.D.,N.D.

In her brave book *The Cure for All Diseases*, Hulda
R. Clark, Ph.D., N.D., explains to us that all diseases
are caused by two things: toxins and parasites.
Toxins accumulate in a certain part of the body and
in the presence of these toxins parasites love to make
their home. If you have ever had a live blood
analysis you have seen parasites inside and in
between your red blood cells, with the white blood
cells trying to gobble them up. These parasites (tiny
worms or stages of worms, viruses and bacteria)
excrete certain aggressive chemicals that cause
disease in our bodies. In the case of cancer, Dr. Clark
finds isopropyl alcohol to be the substance that
attracts and hosts a certain parasite. If somehow this
isopropyl (rubbing) alcohol has accumulated in, for
example, the liver, the parasite that likes to live in

tissue that is loaded with isopropyl alcohol will nestle itself in there and will excrete a toxic substance that works like a cancer growth factor. It stirs up the tumor process and can, in this case, develop into liver cancer.

Is there any way that we can stop the parasite's destructive work, right now? Dr. Clark writes, "Cancer is so easily cured because it is a parasite-caused disease. Kill the parasite and you have stopped the cancer." Thanks to Dr. Clark, yes we can! With her brainchild, the Zapper, we can kill parasites in approximately one hour. (I told you I have good news!)

She further explains in her book in great detail how to get rid of this isopropyl alcohol that paved the way for the parasites. When you have more time to get into the details of her detoxification program, it is worthwhile to follow the practical guidelines in her book: *The Cure for all Cancers*.

> "I set a goal of 100 cases to be cured of cancer before publishing my findings. That mark was passed in December, 1992. The discovery of the cause and cure of all cancers has stood the test of time .....!" (Hulda Clark)

However, we leave these toxins for what they are, right now, and use the Zapper only to buy us time, because as long as we use the Zapper on a daily base, the parasites have no chance to come back to fire up the cancer process again. So, by using the Zapper, we eliminate an important ingredient in the formation of a cancerous tumor.

How does the Zapper work, you ask. Well, you probably have to step out of your "think-box" for a moment, but, alright here we go.

We have to start by understanding that, since everything consists of tiny particles, everything–and I mean everything, even light–is in a constant state of vibration. Atoms, carrots, air, muscles, viruses and people, all are groups of particles vibrating with a certain speed, or frequency. When I hit a G-major on the piano, the string of that particular tone is made to vibrate, which makes the air around it vibrate, which sets my eardrum to vibrate, etc., until it is registered in my brain as a G-major.

It'll tell your age if you remember the singer Ella Fitzgerald, who, on a TV-program, shattered a crystal glass with just her voice. When she would sing a high note with enough volume, the glass would burst in pieces, because Ella's voice vibrated with exactly the same frequency as the frequency of the glass. This is called **resonance**.

And that is exactly what the Zapper does–not with sound, but with electricity. The Zapper sends a small electric current into the body with the same range of frequency as that of the parasites that behave like stowaways in the tissues of the body (flukes, bacteria, viruses, fungi, etc.).

The knowledge of these frequencies comes from way back in the twentieth century, but the application of it in the form and technology of the Zapper is new. In her book you can even find the technical details of how to build one by yourself with parts from Radio Shack, for approximately twenty-five dollars. It is not that easy, though. I recommend buying one. We were in a *hurry* to get well, remember?

So, you buy a "Zapper" from Dr. Hulda Clark for $150 and you use it every day for as long as your doctor says that you have cancer. The (battery operated) Zapper sends out an electrical impulse to your body that kills the parasite that was mentioned in the previous chapter. This parasite excretes a substance that is a growth factor for cell division. When it has been killed, it cannot trigger this cancerous activity any longer. Use it while you watch TV, snooze, or walk. It clips on your belt. So you see that this first step is pretty easy, although it costs you something. However it may be the best money you ever spent on getting well. The Zapper can be used in the control of many other diseases, so it is an excellent addition to your medicine chest.

The latest model, the "Super Zapper de Luxe," comes with a slot that fits special "smart keys" for cancer, diabetes, asthma, fibromyalgia, etc. When a "smart key" has been put into the slot, the frequency is set even more specifically for the condition that the key relates to.

Another reason why you would want to use the Zapper is that the *direct current* by itself is reported to be effective in causing tumor cell death!

Although no side effects ever were reported, out of precaution the Zapper should not be used by people with pacemakers or by women going through pregnancy.

Chapter 5

The Acid Factor

*"The countless names of illnesses
do not really matter.
What does matter is that they all
come from the same root cause...
too much tissue acid waste in the body!"*
-- Dr. Theodore A. Baroody, MD

More and more voices in the scientific community are being heard that confirm this remark from Dr. Baroody.

Our tissues, whether muscle tissue, brain tissue, nerve tissue or connective tissue all have something in common: the cells, or clumps of cells are enveloped by a fluid that has a transport function. This fluid receives nutrients from the blood and passes them on to the cells. The cells drop their waste products via the fluid back into the bloodstream.

You'll understand that it is of the utmost importance to keep this fluid (let's call it the *milieu*) as clean and pure as we can. The purer and cleaner this milieu is, the better the cells will function; the healthier they will stay. If we allow toxins and acid to accumulate in the milieu, the cells will slowly become diseased and will eventually die.

In 1912 a French scientist, Dr. Alexis Carrel, took a piece of tissue from the heart of a chicken embryo and kept it suspended in a bottle with fluid and nutrients. As long as the temperature and consistency of the fluid was kept constant and clean the tissue stayed alive.

Well, the tissue was kept alive for *more than 34 years;* it outlived Dr. Carrel. The chicken heart eventually "died" when the night clean-up crew accidentally messed with it.

As long as we can keep chicken embryo-cells suspended in a perfect milieu they will stay alive and happy. If only we could do this for the cells of our body, we would live in perfect health until we would die simply of very old age.

In our Western culture with our poor dietary habits and toxins, an acidic lifestyle has developed, the symptoms of which are taking on epidemic proportions. The delicate tissues and fluids inside our body are being used as garbage dumps, with the result that they become more and more toxic and acidic and threaten the existence of our cells.

While this insidious onslaught on our health is taking place, most of us don't even realize what is going on. We have no clue and rely heavily on our medical professionals to keep and get us out of trouble; however, our doctors do not test their patients for tissue-acidity. They do test our blood but this does not tell us much about the health state of our *tissues*. We'll talk about this some more later.

In order to give you a good understanding of the danger of having too much acid in your tissues, we need to get a bit more technical. You need to understand a couple of things to be able to convince yourself or your loved ones that something needs to change in the way we live.

5.1   What is Acid, What is Alkaline?

"Cancer can only develop and survive
in an acidic environment."
-- Dr. Otto Warburg

Let's do a little chemistry. A water molecule (H_2O) consists of two different atoms: an H+ and an OH- atom. Because these atoms have a charge (+ or -) we call them ions. A fluid that is very rich in H+ ions and low in OH- ions we call an **acid**. When it is very low in H+ ions the fluid is called **alkaline** (yes, more OH- ions). Acid and alkaline are opposites.

The point where equilibrium is reached is regarded as neutral. Then there are just as many H+ ions as there are OH- ions.

The balance between acidity and alkalinity is reflected in a term called 'pH'. A low pH reflects a high acidity and a high pH reflects a low acidity. (Yes, read that again, pretty confusing isn't it?)

Maybe this will help: when the pH is low we can say that there is an acid pH. When the pH is high there is an alkaline pH. We find neutrality at a pH of 7.0.

Blood must *always* remain at a pH of 7.4 (slightly alkaline) so that it can transport a healthy amount of oxygen from the lungs to the cells. An acid fluid cannot hold oxygen! Blood maintains the delicate pH balance in our whole body, which is very vital for the health in all of our tissues, fluids and cells. All the cells in our body are slightly alkaline and healthy from the start, but when they slowly become more acid (a lower pH) disease can set in.

The only place in our body where a low pH (high acid) is healthy is in the stomach (stomach acid) and in the bladder. In these two organs we need a high acidity in order to digest our food and to get rid of waste products. All other organs and tissues, like muscles, bone, brains, and connective tissue are supposed to be slightly alkaline. They will stay alkaline if many different conditions are met; however one condition is very important: a proper consistency of *mineral* content. Without minerals we loose our alkalinity and we'll acidify.

When an adequate amount of minerals is in the diet, the body tissues can maintain an alkaline pH of 7.4. However when the diet is depleted of minerals, the body is forced to rob Peter (cells and milieu) to pay Paul (the blood).

The blood *must* stay alkaline or we die! To stay alkaline our blood removes crucial minerals, such as calcium, from the bones, muscles, kidneys, liver, etc., in order to maintain the blood at pH 7.4. This causes these de-mineralized tissues and organs to become acidic and that's bad because tissues that are acidic cannot retain oxygen, which is vital for health and survival of the cells. Too little oxygen creates an environment where cancer can develop, remember?

Now you'll understand why it is so important that we stay alkaline, because in an alkaline environment or milieu cells will find lots of oxygen and consequently cancer will not have a chance there.

Yes, I hear you wonder, are my tissues acid or alkaline? How can I find out? That is an excellent question! It shows you're learning fast and you're on the right track! We're about to do a little test!

5.2   The Litmus Test

How can we determine if our body fluids are acid or alkaline? How can we know in what state our body is? Do we go to the hospital, a laboratory, or to our own doctor's office for this? Is it expensive?

The answers are no, no, no and ...no!

There is a simple test that you can do by yourself, that will tell you in ten seconds what the overall state of your body's pH is. It's called the litmus test. With an inch of litmus paper you can test the pH of your saliva, which can be seen as representative for the overall pH of your body tissues and fluids.

Buy a roll of litmus paper at the health food store; cut off an inch of it. After you have not eaten or drank anything for an hour, suck your mouth dry and swallow a few times. Then pour some new spit on the litmus paper. Don't lick or suck on it, but drop your saliva on the paper.

Make it soaking wet. Within five seconds compare the color of your paper with the colors and numbers on the color chart that came with the Litmus paper. A test-score of 6.5 to 7.5 tells you that your body-fluids are in balance or even slightly alkaline, which is to be preferred. A score below 6.5 indicates too much acid. It may even be lower than 5.0. This is an indication that your body is far too acidic, which is a requirement for cancer. Not good!

Please keep in mind that the Litmus test is *not* a cancer test; it cannot tell if you have cancer or not. It only indicates how acidic or alkaline you are. However, those who have active cancer will find that their saliva pH is very likely at 5.5 or lower.

If you scored 6.5 and higher you're doing well. Keep doing what you're doing. If you have scored 6.5 or lower your body fluids are too acidic and you need to change that.

Almost all of the arthritis patients that I have tested so far have scored between 6.5 and 5.5; so there seems to be a correlation between arthritis and a low pH.

Every cancer patient that I have tested with litmus paper scored 5.5 or lower! This step down to 5.5 does not seem to be a big difference; however a person with a 5.5 pH has ten times as much acid in his/her tissues than someone with 6.5. (That's not ten *percent* more, but ten *times* more!)

I've come across people who are diseased in many ways, using sometimes more than twenty different medications, having a pH of 4.5 and even lower! They test more than *one hundred times* more acid than I do.

In this acidic state your body is continually under extreme stress and is negatively affected in many of its functions. This creates a situation that is very susceptible for many different diseases like cancer, lupus, arthritis, multiple sclerosis, osteoporosis, cardiovascular and heart disease and many more. It is a well-established fact that most degenerative diseases develop in an acidic milieu / environment.

There is a lot of good news in this statement, because it means that if we can keep our body fluids and tissues alkaline, these diseases will have no chance of developing in our bodies. It implies that we can prevent many of the horrible diseases that are going around, simply by keeping our pH at a range of approximately 6.5 to 7.5.

If you have scored lower than 6.5 and maybe even lower than 6.0, or even 5.0, the good news still applies to you. You can change your body's pH back to normal values, after which your body will be able to heal itself of disease, even from cancer.

When your tissues and fluids become alkaline again they will absorb and hold a bigger concentration of oxygen and other vital nutrients for your cells. Your cells will jump at the nutrients and oxygen and restore to health over time.

I have noticed that diabetic people often score an extremely high pH with the litmus saliva test. Many diabetics that I tested scored 7.5 and higher, which of course is very suspicious. I let them test their saliva in a different way, which may be more accurate.

Here it is:

> Take a little lemon juice, or anything that will cause the inside of your mouth to taste very acid and just swish it around in your mouth until your whole mouth tastes very acid. Then spit out whatever you took into your mouth to make it acid and swallow a few times until the acid taste in your mouth has *completely* gone. Now test your saliva with the litmus paper and compare it with your color chart.

What you have done is this: you've challenged the inside of your mouth with acid. Alarmed by the high acidity, your little saliva glands did a counter attack by producing as much alkaline saliva as they could to neutralize the acid. If there is a rich reserve of alkaline forming minerals present in your body, your glands had no trouble in defeating the acid; your litmus paper came out blue and even purple.

But if your alkaline reserves were depleted, your glands did not have the ammunition to fight off the acid overload; your litmus test will come out light green or yellow.So here you have a more adequate tool to check your alkaline reserves.

Again, the litmus test is *not* a cancer test, or arthritis test. It only roughly measures the pH in the body. Many doctors agree that an alkaline state of your body relates to overall health, while high acidity goes together with poor health and disease.

My own observation of approximately eighty cancer patients is that *every* active cancer patient scored below a 5.5 pH.

The only exception to this I have found with a skin cancer patient (with a small basal cell carcinoma). His litmus test still was 6.5, which makes me wonder if skin cancer could be a category of its own. I have also seen people with a pH of 5.5 and even 4.5 and lower who did *not* have cancer. Their state of health however was severely compromised by swollen limbs, arthritic joints, muscle spasms and pain.

Only doctors are allowed and trained to diagnose, so do not go around in the neighborhood telling everybody who tests lower than 5.5 that they have cancer or arthritis.

Every kind of Litmus paper has its own color chart and its own range, so when you buy Litmus paper, do the test only with *your own* color chart.

Now, let's see what you can do to get your pH back up to normal values. How can you get the acid overload out of your body and tune your body back to where it can heal itself? That is what the following sections are all about.

Let's summarize. When the milieu of the cells of your tissues has become too acidic (low pH) you want to restore the balance by adding alkaline (high pH) to the milieu. In a milieu with the right pH (7.4) your cells thrive, they will be able to fight off intruders and they will live a healthy cell life. When your body has rid itself of the acid overload, you *cannot* have cancer any longer! It *cannot* come back as long as your tissues are alkaline! Alkalizing your system is a very important job and very essential to getting rid of an important ingredient for cancer.

Cancer-centers are focused on cutting, burning or poisoning tumors in the hope that they will shrink and disappear. The tumors, however, have a nasty habit of coming back again and again, sometimes with a vengeance.

When you alkalize your body, you are not just eliminating tumors; you are killing cancer!

5.3   Alkalizing by Minerals

"You can trace every sickness, every disease, and every ailment to a mineral deficiency."
-- Dr. Linus Pauling, winner of two Nobel Prizes

We mentioned already that to stay alkaline we need a large alkaline *reserve* in the body in the form of minerals. The molecules of minerals are the "carriers" for alkalinity.

Several people groups on earth enjoy remarkable health and longevity: for instance the Hunzas of North Pakistan. Most of these healthy people live high in the mountains, where they drink their water straight from the glaciers.

During thousands of years the glaciers pulverized the rocks trapped at the bottom to rock-dust by the weight of the sliding ice mass. The melting water carried the dust into the rivers downstream coloring them white by the high content of minerals.

Looking at their health, the common denominator of these people-groups is their consumption of incredible amounts of minerals, especially calcium, and trace minerals, which far exceeds (a hundred times!) our American required daily allowance (RDA) that our medical establishment tells us to take. Cancer as well as other degenerative diseases that are rampant in the U.S. are unheard of in these people groups. So there is an important connection between taking in enough minerals and being healthy and cancer-free.

We too will have to consume enough alkaline forming minerals, like calcium (Ca), potassium (K), magnesium (Mg), and sodium (Na), of which calcium is the most abundantly available in the body. Besides these we need minute amounts of "trace" minerals with exotic names like rubidium, germanium, lutetium and many others.

Since the soil used for our agriculture is more and more being depleted of these important substances we find less of them in our foods like vegetables, fruits and grains (bread). Taste for example a tomato from a supermarket and then one from a produce place. You will notice the difference.

The tomato from the produce place tastes saltier and just plain better.

The researcher and author, Bob Barefoot, on one of his audio tapes, tells about exciting tests that were done with a cancer tumor. The tumor was surgically taken out and cut in half; one half was put in a beaker with a saline solution (a solution that resembles our body fluids), the other half was put in a beaker with the same fluid, with a little calcium added. The tumor in the beaker with no calcium kept on growing; however the tumor in the fluid with the added calcium started shrinking. The calcium changed the fluid into a more *alkaline solution,* which stopped the tumor from growing and it started "shrinking."

> Alkaline-forming minerals, in particular calcium, play a crucial role in keeping body fluids and tissues alkaline, which in turn, causes cancer tumors to shrink.

Dr. Carl J.Reich, M.D., had found this beneficial use of calcium already in the 1950s and he saw many of his cancer patients as well as patients with all sorts of other diseases become well again after they reversed their calcium deficiencies.

As you will see in the chart below, calcium is the mineral that is most present in the body, so we will want to make sure to consume plenty of calcium on a daily basis.

Acid Forming Minerals:		
Phosphorus . . . .(P)	670 gram
Chlorine . . . .(Cl)	112 gr
Sulfur . . . .(S)	85 gr
Iodine . . . .(I)	0.014 gr

Alkaline Forming Minerals:		
Calcium (Ca), ...	1,160 gr
Potassium (K)	150 gr
Sodium (Na), ...	63 gr
Magnesium (Mg)	21 gr
Iron (Fe).	3 gr

(The most important minerals per gram in a 154 lb adult man: according to Arthur Guyton's "Medical Physiology")

In the last couple of years much is being said and written about calcium, mostly in relation to osteoporosis. Yes, calcium is making headlines! However, the complete story of how calcium gets into your bloodstream and cells doesn't reach the people who really need to know. Often we are only told half-truths. Let's spend a little time on the absorption of this important mineral that can save our lives.

In nature, calcium always buddies up with another mineral: magnesium. Most calcium tablets come with the necessary magnesium. After calcium has been swallowed and has entered into the stomach, it needs to be ionized, or, in English: it needs to be broken down into tiny bits to become soluble in water. Only then will it be bio-available (available for cell intake).

To *stay* ionized further down in the intestines, the calcium ions in the stomach need to be attached to an acid, the kind that you will find in apple juice (malate), in citrus fruit (citrate), or in milk (lactate), or as calcium-gluconate. Without these acids only a small amount of the calcium can be made available for digestion further down in the intestines.

Having arrived in the intestines, the calcium needs to cross a membrane to be absorbed into the bloodstream. This will *only* happen when vitamin D is present in this membrane. Without vitamin D there will hardly be any absorption of calcium. Vitamin D is made in the skin by sunlight. Please read more about vitamin D's cancer fighting abilities in Chapter 12: "Do's and Dont's."

So on its way to the bloodstream, calcium needs assistance from malate, citrate, gluconate, or lactate to stay soluble, and from vitamin D to pass into the bloodstream. So now you have a more complete story. Just popping calcium tablets is not going to help you much. You need calcium plus magnesium, plus an acid, as well as vitamin D. And after you've done all the right things it is helpful to realize that *only some thirty percent* of all the calcium you're taking will be absorbed and will end up in the circulation. And that only on a real good day!

So where do we find calcium? Like people and animals, plants need calcium to live. Through the roots, plants draw calcium from the soil to make it available not only for their own cells, but their intake of minerals makes them bio-available for animals and people as well. Dark green leafy vegetables are the most natural source of calcium. Even the simple grass that's eaten by cows is a rich store of calcium. Plants should be our number one supplier of calcium.

Although cow-milk is a good source of calcium, the consumption of the milk we buy in the supermarkets has become very controversial. Among many other things, milk contains calcium *and proteins*. Although calcium, being an alkalizing mineral, is beneficial to the body, the milk *proteins* can become an acidifying factor for a body that already has an acid pH. When proteins are metabolized they leave an acid ash or residue, which in a *healthy* body can easily be balanced by the body's available alkaline. The abundance of alkaline will balance out the acid.

In a body that is too acid already, these proteins will cause an even further drop in pH. And when that happens calcium is used to *neutralize* the acid and we probably end up *losing* more calcium (through the kidneys) than gaining. Besides the proteins, the lactic acid in the milk could be another factor in the overall pH drop. Most people who have a low pH tend to not like milk. Since lactic acid in milk makes them even more acid, they have a natural dislike of it. If your pH is below 6.5, you may want to stay away from cow milk. **Goat milk,** if you can get it, has fewer proteins in it and resembles human (mother's) milk.

When your pH is 6.5 or higher, cow milk may be an easy calcium supplier for you. Drink it as raw milk as much as possible since homogenized milk seems to be a cause of heart disease. (The homogenizing process turns the fat in the milk into microscopic little balls that, after being processed by the liver, can damage the walls of the arteries and result in heart disease, according to author Karl Loren!)

Natural sources for other alkaline minerals are: bananas, potatoes, orange juice, raisins, tomatoes, most fruits and most vegetables like broccoli and spinach. They contain lots of potassium, magnesium and calcium. Eat some of them every day if you can and get them from a produce place.

Ocean or sea algae and kelp are a rich natural source of minerals and trace minerals. Ocean water is full of minerals. Anything that grows in the ocean can be an important source of minerals for us.

For a person diagnosed with cancer, who has found him or herself to be too acidic, vegetables and fruits alone are not going to cut it. You'll need to *supplement* with every available alkalizing mineral, food or substance you can get your hands on (in the right doses of course).

On the next pages you will find different ways to alkalize your system back to normal values. Read through this list and find out what will work best for you. If you have been diagnosed with cancer you cannot be too picky and you will want to choose those options that will *really* make a big difference and a fast turnaround.

Calcium is produced in dozens of different kinds of pills, liquids and capsules. Don't get discouraged in front of the rows and rows of minerals and vitamins in the drugstore. Remember the "Note on Calcium-absorption," read the labels, and ask questions. Always make sure your calcium comes with the right ingredients: an acid and vitamin D.

There are several kinds of **coral calcium** on the market (one is endorsed by Bob Barefoot from the TV infomercials). Most come with the necessary acid and the vitamin D as well as trace minerals and other vitamins. Coral calcium is also an ocean product. In his book "The Calcium Factor," Barefoot advises patients who are too acidic to take nine coral calcium capsules each day, three in the morning, three at lunch and three at night.

If coral calcium is not available, or too expensive, Barefoot suggests using plain **calcium/magnesium** tablets in the following way:

- When your pH is in the healthy range (7.5 - 6.5) use Calcium / Magnesium pills with a total weight of 1200 / 700mg, with Vitamin D/A capsules of 2400 IU's / 30000 IU's, daily. (= 6 capsules)

- When your pH is 6.5 - 6.0, use Calcium / Magnesium pills with a total weight of 2400 / 1380mg, with Vitamin D/A capsules 4800IU / 60000IU (12 tiny caps), daily.

- When your pH is 6.0 – 4.5 (or lower) take Calcium / Magnes. pills with a total weight of 3600 / 2070 mg with Vitamin D/A 7200IU / 90000IU (18 tiny caps), daily. (From Bob Barefoot's book: *The Calcium Factor*)

(The IU's stand for International Units. Do not let the numbers intimidate you; the IU's are very, very small amounts.)

Divide the daily intake over the three meals and take the calcium/magnesium with a glass of apple juice or orange juice for the necessary acids.

In 1984, Keith Brewer, (PhD in Physics) and H. E. Satori treated thirty patients with various forms of cancer, using cesium chloride coupled with a high pH diet. All of the thirty patients survived. We would expect the media to be all over this newly found treatment of cancer. The cancer societies could have heralded 1984 as the "year of victory." The various foundations would have aimed their grant-money at further research and development of Cesium as a final cancer cure, we all could have put cancer behind us, and I would not have to write this book.

Well, the reality is that we have to look hard to find *any* research papers at *all* about Cesium. The pharma-comps were not and are not interested!

If you have active cancer right now, you're going to love the next statement:

Cesium is an element with three powerful properties:

- It selectively finds and kills cancer cells
- It eliminates pain
- It works fast

Cesium taken in the form of cesium chloride is like dropping a bunker buster bomb. The large molecule is rapidly absorbed by any cell in the body that is cancerous. Only cancer cells will take in high amounts of cesium chloride. Once inside the cell it cannot get out anymore and raises the pH to a high 8.1 level, which will neutralize the lactic acid that causes pain and forces the cancer cell to die in just a few days. (There is that good news again!) The remains of the dead cancer cell is gobbled up by our white blood cells and disposed of.

Since cesium chloride crosses the blood – brain barrier it is just as effective in fighting brain tumors as tumors in the rest of the body.

Cesium chloride is not sold in most health food stores, so you'll have to shop around for this one on the internet. It comes in tablets of different dosage. A therapeutic dose is at least three grams per tablet and should not be taken for longer than thirty-three days.

Cesium chloride in liquid form is preferred, since it is bottled together with potassium and other trace minerals. The liquid form is simply much more bio-available. One bottle is a month's supply.

After taking cesium chloride for a month the cancer cells are expected to have died. An extended use of cesium chloride is not recommended since it now will become available to and be absorbed by *healthy* cells and you do not want your healthy cells to die!

When taking cesium chloride it is necessary to supplement with at least one hundred milligram of potassium. A banana per day will do. (Five hundred milligram of Potassium per banana.)

The famous German doctor Hans Nieper (1928 – 1998), who used a cesium chloride protocol in Hanover, Germany, has been reported to say: "You wouldn't believe how many FDA officials or relatives or acquaintances of FDA officials come to see me as patients in Hanover. You wouldn't believe this; or directors of the AMA, or ACA, or the presidents of orthodox cancer institutes. That's the fact."

Germanium is necessary for a healthy flow of oxygen in and to the tissues, which improves stamina and endurance. Germanium also has anti oxidant properties.

When the researcher Karl Loren's wife Bonnie contracted cancer of the esophagus he did everything he could to save her. During their struggle he posted his protocol on the internet and his wife recovered. The main ingredient he used was germanium (at least two grams per day).

It is not easy to find guaranteed pure germanium and it is pretty expensive if you buy it in powder form. There is also germanium in solution, sold per bottle.

Sodium can also be taken to alkalize the body. Ask your health-food store owner to give you pure salt (sodium chloride) or better: sea salt, instead of the regular table salt that has aluminum as an additive – and just add a little more salt to your diet.

An even better way is to ask your pharmacist to make a mixture of two parts sodium chloride and one part potassium chloride to be used as salt. In this way the delicate sodium/potassium balance in your body is not disturbed.

Or take half a teaspoon of baking soda in water (sodium bicarbonate) at bedtime, with a banana for the potassium. Ask your health professional about your sodium intake; some people are restricted in their salt intake. Whichever way you choose, make sure you drink plenty of water.

5.4   Alkalizing by Food

From a *prevention* point of view, the best thing you can do to stay healthy is...to eat healthy! The right food choices will greatly help to keep your tissues at a constant alkaline pH level, which keeps cancer and a host of other diseases away.

For those of you who have been diagnosed with active cancer it is a different story. Wouldn't it be great if you could simply eat your way back to health by sticking to a certain diet?

When we talk about our overall intake of daily food, there is no "silver bullet" diet that will knock out tumors or neo plasmas. Dr. Arthur B. Robinson has done research on mice and found that once a cancer has become established, poor diets *decrease* the growth of tumors but healthy diets *increase* the growth rate of a tumor. Translating this research from mouse-health to people-health we may conclude that when we have cancer and we change to a more healthy diet, the tumor starts to thrive as well. What a bummer. Like a parasite a tumor draws strength from your strength!

So what to do? Eat a very poor diet, or starve yourself to kill the tumor? But that would weaken your own immune system as well. Let's try to make some sense out of this.

In 1976, at the age of 42, Dr. George Malkmus was told he had colon cancer. He decided to not follow the road of orthodox medicine and started to read the Bible for guidance on this issue. After a while Dr. Malkmus came to the conclusion that it was his poor diet that had paved the way for the colon cancer. He changed his diet to a strictly vegetarian, raw diet of fruits, vegetables (juice) and nuts, which he later called the *Hallelujah Diet*.

When I saw him 20 years later during one of the many lectures he gives about healthy eating, he looked to me like an example of health and fitness. When he asked the audience that night how many people had 'cured' them-selves of cancer by just eating his Hallelujah Diet, a number of hands went up. Then he asked about people who had recovered from arthritis, multiple sclerosis, lupus and other diseases and again many hands went up.

Dr. Malkmus did not change his diet to a *slightly* better diet. He did not just add a few minerals and vitamins to his former, lousy diet. He went *all the way* and brought his colon cancer to a grinding halt.

We can conclude from this that tumors start in a body that is run down by a very poor diet. When a better or more nutritious diet is followed the tumor benefits from this as well. It will thrive and continue to grow. However when a "perfect" diet is applied the tumor and the cancer-process will throw in the towel, shrivel up and die.

Perhaps you will still say: there is no perfect diet. And maybe you're right. But as you see, for many it paid dividends to go as natural and vegetarian as possible. We're not 'just' talking about weight loss here! We're talking about getting rid of the most dreaded disease on earth, cancer, and listening to the many stories of people who have literally eaten their way back to health. It's do-able!

A number of books have been written about foods that help to alkalize our system. I've done the foot work and gleaned the following directions on foods. On the next pages you'll find in the left column the foods that leave an acid ash and will further acidify the body; the right column consists of foods that will help to alkalize the body.

Foods that are strong alkalizers or strong acidifiers are printed in bold print to help you pick the best alkalizers and to leave out the worst acid-formers. The taste of the food is not an indicator if a food will leave an acid, or an alkaline ash. For example, lemons taste very acidic, however the residue that is left after having metabolized the lemon juice is very alkaline, so lemons produce an alkaline ash in the body.

Acid-Forming Cereals:	Alkaline-Forming Cereals:
doughnuts, dumplings, Grape Nuts, macaroni, spaghetti, noodles, oatmeal, pies and pastry, rice, Cream of Wheat	green, fresh corn

Acid-Forming Dairy Products:	Alkaline-Forming Dairy Products:
butter; all cheese; cottage cheese; cream; custards; ice cream; all boiled, cooked, or dried milk	acidophilus; buttermilk; raw milk from human, cow or goat; whey; yogurt

Acid-Forming Beverages:	Alkaline-Forming Beverages:
liquor, wine, beer, coffee, caffeine-drinks, all black teas, artificially sweetened soft drinks.	Natural Fruit-juices, vegetable juices, like noni-juice and MonaVie Herbal Teas.

Acid-Forming Fruits	Alkaline-Forming Fruits
,cranberries, plums, prunes, and all sugared, or glazed fruits (canned, jellied or preserved) green tipped bananas, green pickled olives and cranberries	apples, apple cider, apricots, avocados, (speckled) bananas, berries, breadfruit, **cantaloupe**, cherries, **dates, figs**, grapes, grapefruit, guavas, kumquats, **lemons**, **limes**, loquats, **mangoes**, **melons**, nectarines, olives (sun dried), **papaya**, passion fruit, peaches, pears, persimmons, pineapples, pomegranates, raisins, tamarind, tangerines, tomatoes

Acid-Forming Nuts	Alkaline-Forming Nuts
nuts (more so if roasted), coconut	**almonds**, roasted chestnuts, dried coconut, dried peanuts

Acid-Forming Meats:	Alkaline-Forming Meats:
all meats, fowl, fish, chicken, beef, shell fish and gravies	only blood and bone

Acid-Forming Vegetables:	Alkaline-Forming Vegetables:
asparagus tips, white beans, brussels sprouts, garbanzos, lentils, rhubarb.	vegetable broth, artichokes, asparagus, bamboo shoots, green beans, lima beans, string beans, sprouts, beets, broccoli, red and white cabbage, carrots, cauliflower, chard, chayote, chicory, chives, collards, cowslip, cucumber, dandelion greens, dill, dock green, eggplant, **endive, escarole,** garlic, horseradish, kane, **kelp,** kohlrabi, leek, legumes (except peanuts and lentils), lettuce, mushrooms, okra, onions, oyster plant, **parsley,** parsnip, peppers, potatoes, pumpkin, radish, sauerkraut (lemon), **seaweed,** sorrel, soy beans, spinach, squash, turnips, water chestnut, **watercress**

Acid Forming Condiments:	Alkaline Forming Condiments:
ketchup (processed), mustard, nutmeg, soy-sauce (processed), vinegar (white and processed)	**agar-agar, cayenne pepper,** garlic, herbs, homemade ketchup and mayonnaise, vanilla extract, yeast.

Miscellaneous Acid-Forming	Miscellaneous Alkaline-Forming
artificial sweeteners, all alcoholic beverages, barley malt syrup, **beer** candy, cocoa, chocolate **cola's, coffee** and **caffeine-drinks,** cosmetics, dressings and sauces, most **drugs,** aspirins, eggs (the white), ginger, jams and jellies, flavorings, **liquor,** marmalade, preservatives as: benzoate, sulfur, salt, brine smoke, sago (starch), soda-water, **sugars** processed from beet or cane.) tapioca (starch), **tobacco** (juice, smell and smoke), vinegar, lack of sleep, overwork, **worry**	alfalfa products, dried, unsweetened Ginger, Honey, Brown rice syrup, Kelp, most herbal teas, yeast cakes. raw, un-pasteurized, apple cider vinegar, sweet brown rice vinegar

The rule of thumb of eating healthy is the 75/25 rule. Try, gradually, to change your eating habits to consuming 75% alkaline foods and 25% acid-forming foods. When you are used to only eating "junk" food, you should not go "wide open" and start eating raw food the next morning. Your body cannot handle it. Gradually shift from cooked food to less cooked food and then to more raw foods, to slowly get your stomach used to your new eating habits.

A wonderful help is the use of a "Juicer." This kitchen machine crushes and mills the raw fruits and vegetables, separating the juice from the pulp. The pulp is thrown away, and, after drinking, the juice does not need to be broken down in the stomach and can easily be absorbed into the bloodstream, to be delivered at the cells' doorstep.

Gradually replace your cooked food with juiced fruits and vegetables. (It is better not to take fruit juice at the same time as vegetable juice since we need different digestive enzymes for each of them.) A juicer is probably the most important "medical device" that you can have in your kitchen! When you plan to buy one, make sure it is a slow turning juicer! The knives of a fast turning juicer heat up the juice and can destroy the beneficial enzymes.

Avoid eating over-ripe fruit; the fruit is full of molds that can overwhelm your immune system. Check your bananas and grapes for brown spots.

Do not drink shortly before or during meals. You dilute the digestive juices, needed for proper digestion.

Do not consume melons or milk with any other foods. They are best digested alone.

> If I were asked, "what is the first major cause of acidosis?" I would have to say: "incomplete digestion!"
> -- Dr. Darrell L. Wolfe AC, PhD

Many elderly people have an undiagnosed problem that can lead to severe underlying physical problems; they do not produce enough gastric juices (stomach acid)!

Remember, the stomach is one place in the body where we do want to have strong acid. Too little acid in the stomach results in poor digestion. To help your body digest the food better, some doctors advise their patients to take a teaspoon of apple cider vinegar in a glass of water with some honey just before you start eating. The acid of the vinegar helps the gastric juices to get the job done. Try this out also when you suffer from general indigestion or heartburn.

Once the food travels from the stomach into the duodenum, it needs to be prepared for absorption into the bloodstream. For this to happen properly the body needs to make many different digestive enzymes that help to break the food down further into tiny bits to pass through the walls of the blood vessels. A shortage of these enzymes results in not being able to absorb the nutrients from the food you're taking in. You eat enough but you don't gain weight. If that is you, ask your health-food store owner for digestive enzyme supplements!

In our American culture people eat far too much meat (beef, pork, poultry, fish, shellfish). Meats have a high content of acid-forming minerals, like *phosphor* and *sulfur* and they're also rich in proteins. We need proteins, but not too much of them. Here's why. When proteins are being metabolized in the body they leave an acid ash that will acidify the body. Not wanting to poison the blood with it, the body will dump the acid via the kidneys into the bladder, which can only take so much acid. This acid needs to be neutralized by a strong alkalizer: calcium, which, if it is not readily available, will be drawn from the bones and cause osteoporosis.

Too much calcium in the bladder can cause kidney stones. A four-double whammy: high acid, calcium depletion, bone loss, and kidney stones all can be caused by eating too much meat-protein!

The Atkins diet and other diets suggest a high intake of proteins to avoid filling up with carbohydrates and gaining weight. "You can eat as much proteins as you want," they say, and sure enough, you'll lose weight! However, in the long run it may be a type of diet for which you pay a high price.

Dr. T. Morter, who has written extensively about the acid alkaline balance, suggests not to eat more meat than the equivalent of a deck of cards per day and that includes your slice of meat on your sandwich! The only protein diet product we've heard about, that alkalizes at the same time, is "Alka-Slim" from Dr. T. Morter.

Obesity is rampant in America. Why? Darrell L. Wolfe (Ac, Phd) has the following theory: since it is a fact that fat-cells store away acid, obesity and cellulites may be ways in which the body stores the acid far away from vital organs. The more acidic you become the more fat cells need to be formed to stack away the dangerous acid! Consequently, re-alkalizing your body may be the best way for you to lose weight!

Lastly, after looking at the food lists, you may want to say: "But you don't understand; I have these cravings for super gulps of diet Coke, doughnuts and hotdogs. I cannot survive on just salads or broccoli!"

Oh really?

Is your body really craving for more phosphoric acid from the Coke and for more artificial sweeteners like Aspartame?

Well, let's see; when your body craves it tells you that it needs *nutrients* and you have only given it things like acid and sugar.

You can eliminate your cravings or hunger pangs with a doughnut and a diet Coke or another soda in the morning, but you are feeding your body only "empty calories". These "empty calories" are fueling your body all right but they do not give you the necessary vitamins, minerals and other nutrients your body also needs for the fueling process. So two hours later you have these cravings again and you down another Coke, and another, and another... I have visited many people with cancer and severe arthritis or other diseases, who drink a gallon of diet soda per day and ask me why they feel so bad.

Physically, your body craves nutrients like vitamins, minerals, essential fatty acids, healthy oils, etc. Let's start giving it what it really needs and you'll see that you do not need all that garbage. You'll probably drop some weight as well.

Cravings can also come from another source: the psyche.

Food cravings are mostly a physical response to being frustrated or anxious. When living under stress some people bite nails, some folks smoke, some go and work out, some even use drugs. Many people in America have learned to use food as a pacifier when they feel overwhelmed by the pressures of life, or when negative emotions are surfacing. The bad feelings are muffled by the wonderful sensations from the taste-buds.

Instant pleasure compensates only temporarily for unresolved frustration!

If this is you, please read on, because you'll find a very effective way to deal with cravings, anxiety, anger, worry and other negative emotions in the following chapters. You'll be delighted to see how easy it is to get rid of life-long hang ups on food cravings and other dilemmas.

By now, you are using your Zapper daily to put your cancer on hold. You're taking in copious amounts of minerals to alkalize your body back to health and you're changing your eating style from inhaling junk food to eating real food: fruits and vegetables. Meanwhile, on a cellular level, you are destroying tumors and you are revitalizing your cells by giving them the nutrients they need. Good job!

You're doing great!

Put your seat belt on and head for the next chapter.

> **WARNING**
> When you are treated for a disease by a physician and take medications, please realize that some of these medications (like Coumadin, or Warfarin), are very sensitive to any sudden change in diet. Inform your doctor if you plan to change to a more healthy diet so he or she can monitor you!

5.5 Alkalizing in a Hurry

In this section you'll find some products that are known specifically for their fast alkalizing action.

• **Cesium chloride.** We have previously talked about this mineral already. Within thirty days you can alkalize your tumor cells and selectively kill them.

Let me try to say this gently in another way:

> This stuff kills cancer cells
> in 1 month!!

When I tell people about this they nearly always stare at me like a rabbit caught in the headlights.

Hello...! Yes, even tumor cells inside the brain!

• **Microhydrin.** As this book goes to print, a new substance is being hailed as a formidable alkalizer and a super anti-oxidant: microhydrin.

This stuff is powerful, folks! It is a product of cutting edge technology!

A top-notch scientist and inventor, Patrick Flanagan, found a way to add an extra electron to the hydrogen ion. These tiny little charged H- ions (H minus ions) bring a load of alkalinity (= electrons) inside the body, while at the same time functioning as anti-oxidants, undoing the damage of free-radicals. One glass of orange juice with one capsule of microhydrin powder mixed in is equivalent in electron power to ten thousand glasses of organic orange juice! What a product!

It is sold as a food and Flanagan claims that the consumption of microhydrin speeds up the alkalizing process from six months to *three weeks*!

Just what we need. A fast way to get rid of acid and to kick cancer in the teeth! Thank you, Doctor Flanagan!

Microhydrin is sold in three hundred milligram capsules and as bulk powder. Find it on the Internet. A similar product with the same formula as microhydrin, but cheaper, is **Hydrogen Boost**, which comes in five hundred milligram capsules.

HydraCel is another great product of Dr. Flanagan's genius. It's a high pH fluid, two drops of which in a glass of water will alkalize the water to a normal value. However, it does more than that. A few drops of HydraCel will also neutralize the toxic chlorine that is in our drinking water and it will change the surface tension of the water to where the water is much better absorbed by the cells.

You can carry this little bottle of HydraCel in your purse or pocket and use it whenever you drink something. (There are more products like this that can be used to alkalize your drinking water, like Ox-E-drops, which are based on sodium chlorite, or Alkalife. I found Ox-E-drops in a local pet store.)

• **MonaVie.** A fruit drink with an extreme amount of anioxidants. MonaVie consists of 30% of the juice of the famous Acai berry. More about this drink in chapter 9.

• **Magnetic sleeping pads.** Yes, you can alkalize your system while you sleep! There is enough science backing up the idea that a magnetic field has an alkalizing influence on the body. The north pole polarity of a magnetic sleeping or seat pad or mattress will encourage the body to become more alkaline. The Nikken company, e.g., sells magnetic sleeping pads and seat pads through independent distributors.

For those of you who can spend plenty of money, there are some innovative and exciting machines out there that are promising in cancer treatment.

• For instance: the **Papimi machine,** which works like a microwave oven that can be used for human tissues since it does not generate heat. When a cell is diseased the electrical potential of the cell wall is depleted. The transport function of the cell wall now has been compromised; it is harder for nutrients to enter the cell and waste disposal slows down.

The inventors of the Papimi machine claim that treatment with the machine will restore the electric potential of the cell walls to normal values in a very short time.

I know personally of an elderly gentleman around eighty years old who had surgery of the intestines. When the doctors found him to be full of cancer they stitched him back up and told him to go home and die "with dignity."

Well, his family members stuck their heads together and, since they had nothing to lose, decided to take matters in their own hands. They agreed about several alternative approaches (all of them you can read in the book you're holding), took their dad home and gave him the "works". Several months later I heard that Dad was doing fine and that he was up and about again. I was told that his overall wellbeing improved significantly after using the Papima machine. Again, the device is designed to restore the missing electrical charge in the cells in order for the cells to overcome their low energy state. Low energy is synonymous with a high acid state.

A similar device is the **REHATRON™alpha**. The FDA has only allowed these machines to be used in the treatment of chronic pain patients. Let's hope cancer patients will be able to use this machine in the very near future.

• **The e-lemon-iser.** Here is an excellent, healthy and simple make-it-yourself drink that helps to alkalize your body.

> - take a gallon jug and pour in purified water,
> - add the juice of 5 squeezed lemons (lemon juice, although it has an acid taste, is a strong alkalizer),

- sweeten it up with grade A maple syrup,
- carefully add the hottest kind of cayenne pepper
  (another strong alkalizer) to this beverage.
- shake well and drink it all through the day.

Dr. L. Horowitz recommends this drink in combination with fasting, although fasting is not a requirement when alkalizing your body. I tried this beverage myself and just could not stand the cayenne pepper.

If you are very sensitive to the pepper you can avoid the burning of your mouth by taking cayenne pepper capsules (health-food store). In this way you can bypass your taste buds. Take the cayenne with your meals (1 to 2 capsules per meal). Start with just one and work your way up. Or, pour a tablespoon of fresh lemon juice in a glass of water and drink one every half hour. This also helps against kidney stones.

• **Vegetable juices.** Also, fresh vegetable juices have a pH of 8.0, drink them instead of the bottled fruit juices that have added sugar.

5.6   Alkalizing by the Mind

This section will answer many questions that spin and tumble around in your brain and keep you awake many a sleepless night, wondering why certain negative things and habits are so hard to get rid of.

No book on health is complete without an attempt to find out what the influence of the mind is on our health. Many books have been written about the psychological make up of cancer patients and about the question if there is something like a "cancer-personality." However, most of the conclusions in these books leave us out in the fog and do not give us practical answers that can help us when cancer has already become a part of us.

Although psychology has been called a science, the exploration of the human mind and spirit go far beyond the empirical limits that have been set for science. So let us skip over a mountain of psychological theorizing and get right down to where the rubber hits the road.

Can things that are going on in my mind have a direct effect on any of my physical functions? Can my emotions or my thoughts have anything to do with the prevention, growth and development of disease and cancer in particular?

The answer is a loud and clear: Yes! Absolutely!

You may want to shrug your shoulders, smile a little and think: "Yeah, yeah, but I read this book to get rid of my cancer, so let's get on with it!"

Well, stay with me because we're on the right track to get you well again. This chapter may become an eye-opener for you and answer many of your questions that weren't answered in the previous chapters.

Perhaps you've come this far in the book and still wonder how in the world you can be sick. You've done everything right; you eat right and may even be a vegetarian, you drink right, you exercise, you avoid toxins and carcinogens and you never indulge in smoking, drinking, etc. If this is you, this will be your most important chapter!

> Never underestimate the influence of your thoughts and feelings on your physical health!

Neurologically, the mind (thoughts and emotions) forms an electrical circuit with the rest of the body. Thoughts and emotions have a direct electrical/physical effect on the functioning of our body, tissues and cells. Take sadness for example; originating in the mind it can cause fluids to flow from the eyes and can produce severe convulsions of the diaphragm. We call it crying, or sobbing. Joyful thoughts pull up the corners of our mouth, bring tears to our eyes and make us exhale explosively. We call it laughter. These are all mind-body connections.

The impulses can flow from the brain to our muscles, but the activity of muscles can just as well send impulses back to influence the brain.

Laughter is called "the best medicine" for good reason. There are documented cases of patients who literally applied laughter as a therapy and became well again. The movie "Patch Adams" follows a medical doctor who walks around in clown's clothes to cheer up his cancer patients and to let them benefit from the healthy and healing activity of laughter.

Norman Cousins was diagnosed with ankylosing spondylitis (something real bad). With only a few more months to live, he checked himself out of the hospital and moved into a hotel room where he took high doses of two things: vitamin C and laughter (comedy videos)! Slowly he regained the use of his limbs and eventually went back to work. Bob Hope, who should have won a Nobel Prize for laughter, reached a belly-aching one hundred years!

We all know that fear can make the hair of our necks stand up and can make us tremble. Fear will very quickly raise the blood pressure; adrenaline will be pumped into the bloodstream that will increase the contraction-force of the heart and will set many muscles on edge. All can be caused by the sound of breaking glass that made you sit up straight in bed scared out of your wits over a possible break-in by a thief, or even worse a rapist like in the movie you just watched. You hear someone walking up the stairs...the door opens...a shadow fills the room...and then a voice: "Hi honey, sorry I'm late...Did you put that old picture frame outside by the garbage? I just kicked it over..."

Notice that it was just the *fear* that set all of your bodily functions in motion. The "thief" did not do it. The experience itself did not trigger off a higher heart rate; it was the fear of the thief that did it. Your fear! Your emotion! Your mind! The fear quickly caused all these reactions and responses to take place so that, if you were be in real danger, you'd run or kick, scream and defend yourself. This reaction is a healthy survival mechanism. It is called the **"fight or flight-mechanism."**

The same emotion of fear, however, can severely disable and disease us. When the fear lingers on even after the threat has gone and when fear becomes chronic, that's when all the trouble starts.

Let's look again at some of the physical reactions that can come with fear:

- the stomach stops its digestion,
- the feeling of having your stomach tied in a knot,
- the undigested food can be eliminated by throwing up,
- the bowels can empty themselves: diarrhea,
- higher blood-pressure,
- the chills, or a hot-flash,
- increased breathing,
- more adrenaline in the bloodstream,
- raised up muscle tone,
- the hair stands up,
- thoughts go in high gear.

When fear or anger continues to be present in our nervous system over longer time periods of time, these same reactions will also continue to affect us physically.

When the dreaded "thief" ended up to be the husband, the nervous system should quickly calm down again and come back into balance. Some people, however, live with constant fear. Something happened in their lives that triggered fear or anger and the experience was never resolved or reconciled. The reason for the anger, fear or sadness can even be altogether forgotten while the physical reactions have become chronic. It seems like our body never forgets!

So now, although the emotion itself has withdrawn from our awareness, we may end up having high blood pressure for years, even for the rest of our lives.

A continual slight rise of the blood-pressure and a small increase of muscle tension can eventually become a severe drain on our health. A higher muscle tone will produce more lactic acid as waste-product, which adds more acid to our system and gradually lowers the pH. The constant muscle tone also uses up more of our precious minerals, which causes a drain on our mineral supply. More acid and less minerals work together to give us acidosis, which makes us more vulnerable for diseases like cancer. Physically this all can begin to overwhelm our immune system and we may succumb to disease.

We go see our doctor who sends us to a heart doctor for our blood pressure, to a neurologist for our muscle spasms, and to a rheumatologist for our carpal tunnel pain. After talking with every doctor for five minutes; after all the tests have come in and after you have talked again with your doctor for five minutes, a diagnosis is made with the inevitable prescription for one or multiple medications. The *emotion* that caused all these symptoms was never even made part of the equation.

In our every day American life, many of us will daily be overcome by a multitude of fears, and anxieties, like the fear of driving, the fear of the people at our workplace or the school-bully, the fear of not being able to live up to the requirements and expectations of the workplace or of losing our job, and the fear of falling into debt or not being able to pay the bills this week, etc.

There are dozens of daily things we can be afraid of, or angry at, without even realizing it. However, our bodies register all this negative input and will present us with the reactions regardless.

How many people in your social group do you know who have high blood pressure, chronic muscle-pain in the neck, obesity, or who are very susceptible to colds, virus infections and allergies? So, yes, there is a mind-body connection.

Emotions, originating in the limbic centre in the middle of the brain, can have an enormous, long-lasting influence on the body and thus on our health. There are also numerous nerve connections between our conscious mind and our body.

Let's talk for a moment about worrying. Do you ever worry?

Worrying is something we can literally do all day and all night. Worry can have us in its grip for years and years and some people even can be stuck in the worrying "mode" all of their lives. Although worrying comes close to fear, it is not so much an emotion as it is a mindset – a way of responding to life's hectic challenges. And with worry we can also mention hatefulness, resentment, bitterness, rage, revengefulness, anxiety, grief, etc.

Scientists have found that worrying directly triggers a large nerve-bundle that connects the brain with the stomach. It's part of the vagus-nerve that manages much of the involuntary reactions. When this nerve is being activated (by negative thoughts, like worry) it will send a signal to the stomach to activate the production of gastric juices, (the juices that digest food in the stomach) just as it normally happens before you start to eat. The stomach glands faithfully respond to the activation by the nerve impulses and secrete hydrochloric acid into the stomach. This is a very strong acid (stomach acid), specifically produced to digest meat, bread, potatoes, candy, etc.

Worrying triggers the production of stomach acid. There is, however, a big problem: *there is no food in the stomach!* So instead of digesting food, the strong stomach acid has nothing better to do than to start irritating the lining of the stomach, which can result in ulcers, or even burn holes in the stomach, with the typical sign of having a dark (bloody) stool.

The strong acid eventually will be poured into the intestinal tract where it will be neutralized by very alkaline juices. For the production of these alkaline juices we need alkaline-forming minerals.

Now you'll understand how a habit of constant worrying can cause us to become depleted of minerals, resulting in acidosis and the risk of falling pray to diseases like cancer.

More than once I have visited patients who had to be hospitalized for a while and who came home with an upset stomach, which later turned out to be bleeding ulcers of the stomach. Their stay in the hospital was a reason for severe worry and anxiety, twenty-four hours per day, seven days per week. When they came home they worried even more after receiving the hospital bills in the mail.

> Constant negative thoughts or emotions can drain the body of its mineral supply, lower the pH, and make us vulnerable to all sorts of diseases.

Gloria, seventy-four, with a happy-go-lucky character, was told by her doctor that the scanner showed a spot on her right kidney. She had an appointment to see the doctor again a week later to talk about this. All that week she worried if she would have cancer in the kidney. Before all of this happened I had tested her saliva pH with litmus paper. She scored a healthy "blue," around 7.0. However, two days of worrying for the result of the scan brought her pH down to 6.0. She told me how afraid she was of what the doctor might tell her next week. Fear and worry had a grip on her and it showed in her saliva pH.

It is for good reason that the Bible warns us not to worry about tomorrow or to harbor fear, anger, bitterness or hatefulness. Some of the people I've tested with litmus paper told me that they were very careful in what they ate and how much; they hardly ate any meat and liked eating vegetables and fruit. They did all the right things, but still they tested too acidic.

How can that be? Maybe this is you. You know you are doing all the right things to stay healthy. You may even be a vegetarian, but you still score green or yellow with the litmus test.

This is an indication that you have to look beyond your diet and examine yourself for possible negative emotions or negative thinking.

Many of us don't realize how negative our thought-life really is because "stinkin' thinkin'" has become a habit. Just like with smoking: we don't smell the bad odor in our clothes anymore, while other people do. Our daily fears and anxieties can have the upper hand in our lives without us even realizing it. If this describes what is going on in your life at this moment, it is time for a thorough spring cleaning! Open the windows of your mind!

"That is easier said than done," I hear you say. How do you get rid of thoughts or emotions that can be so deeply rooted in your inner man, or inner woman? Even psychotherapists have great difficulty counseling people with fear, anger or worry. And their fees alone are reason enough for most of us to start worrying and chew on our finger nails.

Do we find ourselves in a dead end street or is there a way out of the strangle-holds of negative emotions and "stinkin' thinkin'"? Yes, there is, but before this practical way out is introduced, we first have to look at a human attribute that is strong enough to clear up most negative emotions: forgiveness.

Most negative emotions can be traced back to a messed -up relationship. Somewhere down our life we all have experienced disharmony with someone we cared for or loved. It's so human! At that moment of conflict a switch on our switchboard was flipped to the "off" position and it will stay off until the problem is resolved and the relationship has been reconciled.

In a perfect world the person who wronged you will return to you, acknowledge his/her guilt and ask you for forgiveness. In that same world you would forgive whatever it was, hug the other person and both of you would live on in restored harmony, forgetting what lay behind you.

In this scenario two persons will benefit. The perpetrator has gotten rid of his/her guilt and the person who was wronged has freed him/her self of feelings of hate and sadness. No more bad feelings. Emotions restored to positive. No further need for continuation of physical reactions. Restoration of health. Besides the two people who had the conflict there are dozens of people in the background who also benefit from this restored relationship. They too will sleep better and receive a health and wellness benefit.

But now I hear you yell: "Whoa, wait a minute... We don't live in a perfect world, buddy. Nobody came to me to say he was sorry!"

You're absolutely right We don't live in a perfect world and nobody is perfect. So here is some problem scenario: You were wronged but nobody shows up to acknowledge his/her guilt or ask for forgiveness.

It is your health that is at stake. When you are suffering from cancer, *you* are suffering from cancer! Your sadness or hatred has a negative influence on your body! In this case you will have to practice forgiveness on a one-sided basis. You'll have to sit down somewhere or to go for a walk preferably in the presence of a friend (God?) and literally speak out forgiveness to such and such. Speaking it into your own ears will do something in your brain and in your spirit that will set you free from hate and sadness, two elements that are acidifying your body.

Please do not make the mistake of thinking that by forgiving a person you justify his wrongdoing. You do not and you can not! The only person who can justify is God. When you forgive a person you do not justify the wrong he or she did to you. You 'only' cancel the debt he or she has with you. On the other side, forgiveness sets *you* free from your pursuit to get even. And it is often this dynamic of "I was wronged and now I must and will get even!" that we carry around with us like a dead corpse. It's heavy and it stinks. The bitterness, anger and rage that come with this, have a very acidifying effect on us and can keep us in a state of poor health for the rest of our lives.

So, your act of forgiveness must not depend on the other person's acknowledgment. It must be *unconditional*. This is a very difficult thing to do and it gets even harder when the Bible tells us to forgive from the heart.

One-sided forgiveness is very hard. However you're in excellent company. God is practicing one-sided forgiveness on a daily, 24/7 schedule.

Here's another bum scenario: You acknowledged your guilt and you asked for forgiveness, but you're given the cold shoulder. This too is frustrating since the relationship is not restored. You will have to determine you own sincerity in this matter and after trying your best there is only one thing to do and that is to let it go. While there is no one to take the blame off your shoulders, you may want to meditate on the following scripture in the Bible: 1 John1: 9: "If we confess our sins, He [God] is faithful and righteous to forgive us our sins and to cleanse us from all unrighteousness."

We humans have a great need to be forgiven! None of us is perfect; we all have made and will make mistakes and by doing that we put a load on our backs that is called guilt. Guilt acidifies the body because it gives us bad feelings and it makes us worry, hate and fear. We were not created to carry guilt around. It kills. So get rid of it! Make up with whoever you have wronged. Ask for forgiveness and/or be forgiven. It is really that simple. Do not allow a relationship-problem to be the cause of your sickness. You'll pay a high price and will carry a heavy burden.

In this context we can see how healthy and beneficial it is if a person has a good relationship with the people around him or her and with God, who is the ultimate forgiver.

Another sublime way to stay in the best of health, to keep your system alkaline and to have healthy relationships is to have an attitude of gratitude.

Earl, at 88 years old, was physically slowing down considerably and showed some functional decline. He was, however, thankful for every little good thing that happened to him and always expressed gratefulness every time I left him after a work-out. When I tested his saliva pH it was 7.0, which, at his age, is remarkable. He died a week later simply of old age, with a prayer on his lips.

A Japanese researcher, Masaru Emoto, started taking photographs of frozen water crystals. He discovered that water expresses itself in a multitude of ways.

When exposed to beautiful harmonious music, the (distilled) water would form splendid crystals, formed like flowers. However when exposed to the shrieks and dissonants of rock music, water could not even make a crystal. Later he found that, in a similar way, water would form nice and organized crystals when spoken to in a loving way, but when harsh words were uttered in the presence of the water it could, again, make no crystals.

The picture that Mr. Emoto proudly shows off on the front cover of his book: *The Hidden Messages in Water*, is truly the most beautiful of all water crystals. It was taken after water was exposed to two words: love and gratitude!

There is a message for all of us in here. Human bodies consist of more than seventy percent water. No doubt, on a microscopic level, our words and attitudes have an impact on the structure of our water molecules and thus on our physical being. An attitude of love and gratitude will be translated by the water in our bodies into health and wellness, I'm sure.

I love it when the discoveries of scientists on a physical level confirm the *spiritual* truths of the Bible. Once the choice to forgive and to express love and gratitude has been made, mountains of anger, bitterness, fear and worry can dissolve like hail in Florida.

Sometimes, however, this does *not* happen, or not completely. After doing all the above, negative emotions and thoughts can still continue to overwhelm us. Although there is no longer a reason for them to be in our conscience, they can keep harassing our thought life and keep us from sleep.

It's not because we didn't forgive enough, or had a wrong attitude, but because these emotions and thoughts often keep lingering on in our nervous systems, just like a car engine that sometimes can keep running although you have switched off the ignition and taken the key out. The only way to stop the engine then is to lift up the hood and disconnect the battery for a moment. By doing that you "reset" the car's electrical system. In order for us to become free of these freewheeling negative thoughts and emotions we need to somehow "reset" our nervous system.

I'm going to tell you some more fabulous news. There is a fast, cheap and simple, do-it-yourself way to eliminate negative thoughts, emotions and the effects they have on our life. It works much like in the example of the car. Like "resetting" the electrical system of the car, this technique can reset the nervous system of the body.

It is a method I had never heard of before and, if I would have had a bad day, I probably would have pooh pooh-ed it away as nonsense after a good laugh. I became interested in it, however, after trying it out on my lower back pain, and receiving, to my great surprise, an instantaneous result.

The method is called Emotional Freedom Technique (EFT). EFT is a simple technique of tapping with two or three fingers at different places on your body. These places relate to acupuncture points (places of low skin resistance, where the body's energy system can be influenced) and by tapping on them, energy is applied that somehow finds a way to the brain and extinguishes negative emotions or thoughts in our memory.

I have read many impressive results of EFT: from getting over the fear of heights and rats, nightmares, etc, to pain that was relieved within minutes after applying the tapping. More and more professional people are starting to use EFT in their own practice.

Doctor Joseph Mercola has one of the largest medical websites with lots of cutting edge information on health issues with an alternative approach. He treats most of his patients *first* with EFT, simply because it is so effective in the treatment of many different symptoms and conditions.

You will find an extract of the EFT manual in Appendix A, but for now please continue on and we'll talk more specifically about the effects of stress on the body.

5.7 Stress Acidifies

According to the Centers for Disease Control and Prevention up to 90% of the doctor-visits in the USA may be triggered by a stress related illness.
-- USA Today 03-25-05

The much enjoyed pictures of Norman Rockwell are fading away rapidly in our days and even good old Mister Rogers recently passed away; both leaving a legacy of how enjoyable life was and how harmonious it can be.

American life has changed to a culture geared for stress. Most families have to come up with a double income to pay for the life that our television portrays as the "all-American way of life." Many people even work double jobs to make ends meet and in the process of getting there, families break apart into units with single moms or dads.

Work has changed. Scientists and planners have come up with quotas that have to be met. Lawyers force us to cover our backs with endless piles of paperwork. All the responsibilities! All the pressure! All the hurry! And then there are all these bills and payments! Will it ever end?

Stress is anything that forces us out of balance (physically and/or mentally). When we're being pushed, we push back to stay on our feet. This kind of stress is, for most people, a healthy challenge, a challenge that can be handled and overcome in a certain time. It is the kind of stress that puts us on our toes and that challenges us to achieve things in life. There is also a dis-stress. Distress happens when we're being pushed (physically or mentally) either too much or for too long a period of time.

When we are under a healthy stress, we'll recuperate from our exertion in a short time. After a weekend well spent we can face another week in the workplace. Mentally and physically we have come to rest.

However, when we experience distress there often is not enough time to rest and regain our strength, or the rest is not deep enough to replenish our reserves. We do not seem to *fully* recuperate from distress; and slowly but surely the effects of distress can accumulate and overwhelm our physical and mental being. This is why distress also is called **chronic stress.**

Stress switches on the warning lights and alarms in the body and *leaves them on*. Many chemical changes happen in the body to adjust to the alarm situation. Normally all these stress reactions and adjustments are only happening for a short while, but under (chronic) distress the alarms are on continually.

Recently it was discovered that people under chronic stress had above-normal levels of interleukin-6 (IL-6), an immune-system protein that promotes inflammation and has been linked with heart disease, infections, diabetes, osteoporosis, rheumatoid arthritis, and also certain types of cancers.

Chronic stress can weaken a person's immune response, leaving him or her more susceptible to infection, and can lead to unhealthy lifestyle habits. For instance, stress often leads people to overeating, loss of sleep, and neglecting exercise, all of which on their own can create health problems.

In a laboratory experiment, mice were encased and poked with a stick to irritate and provoke them. Upon dissection it was found that all had developed stomach ulcers, some of which had hemorrhaged. An examination of their blood revealed the pH value had dropped by 0.2, clearly indicating that their whole bodies had been highly acidified.

In his book, *The Stress of Life,* Hans Selye writes, "Stress stimulates our glands to make hormones which can induce a kind of drunkenness." Furthermore: *"The fact is that a person can be intoxicated with his own stress hormones"* (p. 412).

While we are under stress, the adrenal glands are "pumping" stress hormones into the bloodstream and, after being used, these hormones are being eliminated by a process called fermentation, which creates a more acid pH in our body. Here too, we encounter our familiar enemy: acidosis.

Chronic stress is just another enemy of our internal milieu, which pulls our pH down to unacceptable low values.

> An imbalanced hormone production will lead to acidification of the tissues, creating a condition for oxygen deficiency in the cells which ultimately results in disease.

How do we keep a tighter rein on distress? Without even making an attempt to give a complete answer, let's focus on some causes that may be overlooked by many folks when it comes to stress. Do not underestimate the effect of all these hormones being used every day and night, leaving us in an acid state.

Physical stress may be the easiest stress to avoid. If our job is physically too demanding, or if the workplace is too toxic, we can find another job in another geographical work-area.

Mental stressors are not so easily identified or avoided. Still, if you take the time to think about it they all seem to revolve around being in debt; or, to use an old fashioned term: being found wanting. And I'm not just talking about money! Something or somebody has a hold or grip on us and we cannot seem to shake it off, probably because the hold is legitimate.

The best example of course is a money debt that, as long as our income comes in steadily, we do not experience as a tight grip on our life. However when for some reason our flow of income has suddenly stopped, the debt can become an enormous stressor. Being conscious we're behind on payments the stress-symptoms begin to introduce them-selves in our lives. We feel we're being strangled...

We can also be in debt in a relationship. When we've sown disharmony in our relationship with another person in any shape or form, we've become guilty of breaking a very simple and common sense rule: love your neighbor as yourself.

Being guilty is being in debt. How? Well, we can owe someone an apology or a visit, or a lunch, or a phone call and if we don't own up to our guilt and redeem it, the guilt will settle in our conscience as an unpaid bill and it may pop up daily in our emotional brain and cause feelings anger, sadness, depression and fear. Many psychologists and psychiatrists will tell you that most mental suffering is generated by feelings of guilt. Many people suffer mentally and ultimately physically because they live under guilt.

We, humans, were not created to live *under* something other than God. As a matter of fact, according to the book of Genesis we were created to live with God.

Guilt is an unbearable burden for humans. Guilt stresses. Guilt makes us sick and guilt kills because it separates us. We were designed to live in harmonious community with each other. When we are in debt, we are out of synch and out of touch.

In the Bible the apostle Paul warns us: "Owe nothing to anyone, except to love one another."

So get out of debt and stay out of debt as much as you can.

Another super stressor is the inability of many people to live in the present; in the now. Think for a moment: all our sadness was caused some-where in the past; all our fears are about things or events that might take place in the future. Our anger was generated in the past. Frustration is created by expectations that were formed in the past or by foreseeing misery that may never come about in the future. Our bosses and schedules tell us to plan ahead and not to forget to write the paper trail of things that happened yesterday.

Although all our daily activities take place in the immediate present (driving a car, typing a letter, walking in the street, etc.), our mind is feverishly occupied with the things that will or may take place in the future (cannot pay the mortgage next week), or that are anchored in the, sometimes, distant past (an un-reconciled relationship with a family member). Meanwhile we do not even realize that we are driving a car, or walking. We can be completely unaware of the now.

I agree this has its benefits, but somewhere in the day our mind, which is in the future or the past, should find its way back to our body that continues on in the now.

How much time do you spend per day being aware of the immediate things or people around you? Have you seen the joggers walking by with their ears plugged up listening to whatever? How long has it been since you walked through a forest and engaged in the light shining through the leaves or stood motionless watching a deer pass by?

Well, you may say: "I'm just not that lucky; I'm working two jobs to get by." Fair enough!

Switch off the TV for half an hour. Walk around the block and focus only on what you hear. Sit in a hot tub and play with the bubbles. Wait for a traffic light and be aware of your neck-muscles. Try to relax them completely. When our mind, our body and our spirit are united again we often experience – wholeness.

I believe we were not created to live here on earth in three different time-spans. We cannot focus on today's business now if we have to drag along the negative things of the past or the fears of the future at the same time.

> As a gift, God gave us the "now" to live in; isn't that why He called it "the Present?"

Could this be the reason why so many people nowadays commit themselves to techniques, like yoga, that force them to, literally, sit down, shut up, and focus on the present, on the here and now?

It is the author's heartfelt belief that, in order to get back in touch with the present, with our body, with nature, with our loved ones and with our creator, we do not have to commit to certain techniques. For us to live in harmony, we only need to find the "place of rest" and live in it. We have to spend more time focusing on the here and now, even on a hectic day when everything seems to go wrong. Rest can be found by reconciling with ourselves, with our neighbor (whoever that may be), and of course with our creator.

This rest (or peace, or shalom) can be experienced in the car, in a hospital bed, in a cubicle, under the shower or on a mountain top. Rest is knowing that it's all right even at a time when life is raging around you at full throttle. God is extending this rest to anyone who really wants it. Rest is perfect harmony.

Dr. T.A. Baroody writes in Chapter 29 of his book *Alkalize or Die*:

> "All emotions, thoughts and feelings, of whatever kind, are felt in the physical body. Those which are inharmonious produce acid reactions."

University of North Carolina researchers studied the stress-response and hormone levels of thiry-eight couples before and after watching an excerpt from a romance film (a *"chick flick"*) followed by a twenty-second hug. This "happy moment" resulted in the following:

- a lowering of the stress-hormones cortisol and norepinephrine,
- a spike in oxytocin, a hormone associated with love,
- the result of these two combined reactions lowered the blood pressure and reduced stress in the subjects.

It has also been found that those people living in happy matrimony have higher levels of flu-fighting antibodies than those who were widowed or divorced.

Stress wreaks havoc on your body! Be smart and de-stress. Do not allow the past or the future to destroy your body in the now.

Get out of debt and stay out of debt. Refuse to live under guilt.

What benefit is it to live in a gorgeous house for which you cannot afford the payments, while you let the place you really live in – your body – deteriorate to a garbage dump?

Chapter 6

The Cell Wall Factor

"Cancer treatment can be very simple and very successful once you know how."
-- Dr. Johanna Budwig

By now you should be pretty excited about the fact that you can actually help your body to push back cancer by simply alkalizing it back to normal values. Are you using the zapper? Did you make changes to your diet? Are you taking minerals?

Well, we are going to eliminate another ingredient in the development of cancer. You'll remember that cancer only can happen when the cell walls have been damaged. The walls that envelop the cell are enormously complex bio-systems. In the walls are openings (gates) that selectively allow nutrients to enter the cell and waste-products to leave. Cancerous cells cannot function properly because, amongst other problems, the "gates" in the walls have lost their selectivity; they let unwanted "intruders" in and leak valuable nutrients out. One type of intruder is the notorious anti-oxidant, which we will discuss in more detail in Chapter 9.

Toxins too can come in and mess with the contents of the cell, like the DNA, which is the substance that directs our natural repair system and keeps us alive. Toxins can cause great problems for the important electrical charge of the cell and for the delicate acid/alkaline balance inside the cell.

The main cause of this wall damage is our intake of hydrogenated fats and oils (margarine, mayonnaise, vegetable oils, etc.).

The building blocks of the cell walls consist of fats. If our body cannot get the right fats to build its walls it has to use whatever is available and the hydrogenated fats make very poor building material!

This chapter is about healing these walls. You are about to find out how many cancer patients have regained their health just by eating a very tasty dessert topped off by a glass of ...Champagne.

Our typical American diet consists of foods that, since the second World War, have been so depleted of nutrients, that sickness and disease have become an almost inevitable consequence. It is shocking to read what the food industry has done to the stuff we put in our bodies daily.

Bread-flour, vegetable oils, noodles, dairy, etc, have been altered to make them look, smell and taste good and give them a long shelf life. However, taking out the essential fatty acids, vitamins, minerals, trace minerals and other vital elements leaves us hardly more than fattening stomach fillers.

According to Dr. D. Rudin, (a Harvard-educated physician and former director of the Department of

Molecular Biology at the Eastern Pennsylvania Psychiatric Institute in Philadelphia):

Compared to 100 years ago, Omega 3 is down 80% and B vitamins are estimated to be down to about 50% of the daily requirement.

Vitamin B6 consumption may be low as it is removed in grain milling and not replaced. Vitamins B1, B2, B3 and E have also been lost in food processing. Minerals are depleted in a similar way. Fiber is down 75-80%.

Anti nutrients have increased substantially: saturated fat, 100%; cholesterol 50%; refined sugar nearly 1000%; salt up to 500%; and funny fat isomers nearly 1,000%.

A *crime* has been and still is perpetrated on the people of the Western countries. The industrialists stole these essential nutrients from our foodstuffs and changed the healthy fats into hydrogenated fats to increase the shelf life of these products. In order to stay healthy, we now have to go to health-food stores to buy these nutrients back and supplement our daily food with them. What is wrong with this picture?

One of those foodstuffs that is missing in our diet is omega 3 fatty acid. A German doctor in bio-chemistry, Dr. Johanna Budwig (nominated seven times for the Nobel Prize) found out that, "healthy people had a much higher content of Omega 3 fatty acids in their blood than those who are ill with cancer (and other diseases)."

Omega 3 is vital for the blood's transport of oxygen. Budwig came to the conclusion that the vast majority of chronic illness is caused, amongst other things, by the improper mass production of oils. (No, the industrialists do not like her!)

Based on her observations, Dr. Budwig started treating patients by giving them a combination of pure flaxseed oil and cottage cheese, which is rich in high quality proteins. By mixing the oil with the sulfur-based proteins, the oil becomes water soluble and more readily available for absorption by the body. The fatty acids can then enter the smallest capillaries, dissolving and cleaning out any of the undesirable fats that the body had to deal with in the past, and bring new life in the form of oxygen. Again, the omega 3 fatty acids give us the right material to build healthy cell walls and they even *replace* the old, unhealthy fats.

But there is more. With the intake of these essential fatty acids you will literally fill your body with new energy. They will bring the charge back into each cell in the form of electrons. The influx of new electrons will have an alkalizing effect on the cell and its surrounding fluids, which in turn will allow more oxygen. Healthy cells will flourish and unhealthy cells will starve.

This oxygenated, healthy, non-acidic environment will, as Dr. Budwig points out in her lectures, knock out the cancer cells.

Following are some statements made by different doctors about Dr. Budwig and her remarkable work.

What she (Dr. Johanna Budwig) has demonstrated to my initial disbelief but lately, to my complete satisfaction in my practice is: **CANCER IS EASILY CURABLE,** the treatment is dietary/lifestyle, the response is immediate; the cancer cell is weak and vulnerable; the precise biochemical breakdown point was identified by her in 1951 and is specifically correctable, in vitro (test-tube) as well as in vivo (real life). — Dr. Dan C. Roehm M.D. FACP (Oncologist and former cardiologist)

Numerous, independent clinical studies published in major medical journals world wide confirm Dr. Budwig's findings. Over 40 years ago Dr. Budwig presented clear and convincing evidence, which has been confirmed by hundreds of other related scientific research papers since, that the ESSENTIAL FATTY ACIDS WERE AT THE CORE OF THE ANSWER TO THE CANCER PROBLEM. You will come to your own conclusions as to why this simple effective prevention and therapy has not only been ignored ...it has been suppressed! — Dr. Willner, M.D., Ph.D. (The Cancer Solution)

In 1967, Dr. Budwig broadcast the following sentence during an interview over the South German Radio Network, describing her incoming patients with failed operations and x-ray therapy: "EVEN IN THESE CASES IT IS POSSIBLE TO RESTORE HEALTH IN A FEW MONTH AT MOST, I WOULD TRULY SAY 90 PERCENT OF THE

TIME." This has never been contradicted, but this knowledge has taken a long time reaching this side of the ocean, hasn't it? Cancer treatment can be very simple and very successful once you know how. The cancer interests don't want you to know this. May those of you who have suffered from this disease (and I include your family and friends in this) forgive the miscreants who have kept this simple information from reaching you for so long — Dr. Roehm M.D, FACP.

How to prepare the "daily dose" of Dr. Budwig's diet: Buy a bottle off **Flax seed oil** (which is very rich in omega 3 fatty acids) from the health food store. (Barleans seems to be a good brand) You should find it inside the store's refrigerator because it has to be kept cool.

Also keep it cool in the car and when you come home put it in the fridge *immediately*. You need one more item: cottage cheese!

Make yourself a bowl (1 cup) of cottage cheese and pour in 4 - 6 tablespoons of flax seed oil. Stir it well, or put it in a blender. While stirring, the oil will disappear into the cottage cheese. You can add some fruits to make it tastier. Optional additions are a little garlic, a little red pepper, or a little champagne. (Yes, a *little* champagne!) Eat some of this mixture at breakfast, at lunch, and at dinner time. The next day you'll prepare a new bowl and repeat what you did the day before. Keep doing this every day for as long as you have cancer.

Once your doctor tells you that you are in "remission", which means that the cancer is gone or dormant (this literally means the cancer is asleep), you can stay on a maintenance dose of one tablespoon of flax-seed oil per 100 lbs of body-weight hot:plus, but :in a cup of cottage cheese.

Yogurt can take the place of cottage cheese, but more of it is needed; actually about three times as much and if fruited yogurt is used it would need to be even more.

Flax seed oil will keep a year in a freezer, four months in a refrigerator, but only three weeks at room temperature.

At *www.whale.to/a/beckwith.html* Mr. Clifford Beckwith tells his story about successfully using flaxseed oil with cottage cheese in his fight against cancer of the prostate and shares the many testimonies of people who followed his example. There are numerous other books and websites from doctors that write about the benefits of omega 3 fatty acids, just search on the internet for omega 3, or flax seed.

Chapter 7

The Oxygen Factor

*"Almost anything can cause cancer,
but, even for cancer, there is only one
prime cause ...the lack of cellular oxygen. "*
-- Dr. Otto Warburg

A lack of oxygen is, as we discussed in Chapter 1, a requirement for cancer development. In 1932 Otto Warburg won the Nobel Prize in Medicine for the discovery that cancer cells are an-aerobic.

Normal cells generate energy from a chain of chemical processes called "the Krebs cycle." Oxygen plays an all important role in this cycle. When there is enough supply of oxygen in the tissues the cell's engines will keep humming steadily. However, when the tissues somehow become depleted of oxygen and the demand for oxygen inside the cell is not met, the cell will change its energy generating program and will start to use sugar as fuel instead of oxygen.

The downside of using sugar is that the cell generates far less energy and leaves more acid as a waste product, which drops the pH of the cell to lower values. This, as you know by now, allows even less oxygen to be present in the cell. Acid expels oxygen, remember! Yes, it becomes a vicious cycle.

By now many changes have taken place inside the cell; it has become a cancer cell and we're on our way to try to reverse this bad situation. Several anti-cancer therapies are focused on trying to starve cancer cells by switching to a non sugar diet, which is hard because sugar is found in many different foods. You do good by keeping your sugar intake as low as you can, but do not starve yourself to the point where you get weak and cranky; you need energy to fight back!

An excellent way to reverse the acidic, oxygen expelling, situation in the cell is to alkalize it, as we've seen in Chapter 5. Alkaline cells suck up the oxygen and where there is an abundant amount of oxygen the cell will change back to its original plan of making energy.

Offering oxygen to an acid cell will not do us much good, since it cannot absorb the oxygen. But if we alkalize the cell first and then supply it with oxygen, it will gladly suck it in and change back into a normal cell. So now that we're doing everything to alkalize our body, let's find out how we can flood our tissues with oxygen.

The first thing we should think about is simply: exercise! Walk outdoors with a quick enough pace to feel yourself breathing deeper and faster for thirty minutes. When coming home, rest for a while and you should feel good.

Do not exercise to the point of over-exertion! Cancer patients have too much acid in their tissues already; they do not need an acid overload from the muscles on top of that. So if you find out that you can only walk for five minutes, then don't do more than that; you'll do better to walk more times per day. For some it will be too much even to go for a walk. Still you can improve your oxygen intake by simply in- and exhaling deeper. While you watch tv, taking several deep breaths with every commercial can give you a significant increase of oxygen.

Do not be discouraged by the "perfect" bodies of athletes and exercise-aholics. It is not the size of your chest or your lungs that defines the amount of oxygen intake in your body. We all have seen the men and women running marathons for the Olympics. They have excellent lungs and highly effective breathing techniques and yet they too have fallen pray to cancer when their bodies became too acidic.

The quality of the air we breathe is of course an important factor. Dr. Kurt W. Donsbach D.C., Ph.D. an expert on the therapeutic use of oxygen, writes,

> "The oxygen content of our atmosphere of a few hundred years ago was about 35%. Today it is 19%".

This by itself is reason enough to make sure we do everything possible to supply our bodies with more oxygen.

There are different therapeutic ways to get a higher oxygen concentration in the body. In the last hundred years oxygen therapies have been successful in the treatment of many different diseases like AIDS, arthritis, and cancer.

Inside the body oxygen is found in different chemical compositions: as O_2 (oxygen), or O_3 (ozone), but also bound to Hydrogen as in H_2O (water) and as in H_2O_2 (hydrogen peroxide).

Therapeutically, hydrogen peroxide (not the one from the drugstore, which is not for consumption; but the food grade kind of hydrogen peroxide!) and ozone can be found in different therapeutic applications; in drinks, crèmes, powders, pills, drops, IV's and in air purifiers.

In the health food store you will find many oxygen products that can be taken orally. Some come as liquids, some as powders and others in tablets. They are all based on "stabilized oxygen," which does not taste as abominable as plain hydrogen peroxide.

I know how bad hydrogen peroxide tastes. Thirty years ago I suffered from a chronic sinus infection. Even after doctors surgically opened up my sinuses, the infection would not leave. I read Ed McCabe's *Oxygen* book and took three to ten drops of 30% food grade hydrogen peroxide in an eight ounce glass of milk, water, or juice. After ten days, my sinuses were well and without infection. Thank you, Ed.

Normal hydrogen peroxide is 3% and has been stabilized with chemicals that are not for human consumption. Food-grade hydrogen peroxide is 30% and dangerous. The 30% will give a burning sensation and a whitish discoloration of the skin when you spill it. Only use it diluted as directed on the bottle. Besides using it in drinks peroxide can also be added to your spa- or bathwater or applied as a body spray in the shower.

Other oxygenating products, some of which have been around since the 1930's, are: Oxy-Dan, Oxy-Max, DynamO2, and Ox-e-drops. (I bought Ox-e-drops at a pet store recently).

They all come in small bottles, but do not underestimate how much oxygen one drop can hold!

Some products split water inside the body into oxygen and hydrogen: Cellfood®, Oxymune®, and Hydroxygen®.

Ed McCabe reports many case histories of people using these products successfully against cancer, AIDS and other viral infections.

By the way, oxygen is one of the few known antidotes against viral infections, so why not load up on some of these bottles and prevent yourself and your loved ones from getting infected by all these new viral diseases that we're being warned for almost daily, like the avian (bird-) flu! Ask your health food store owner! No prescription needed.

Ozone, or O_3, has a history of its own which is recom- mended reading material. As early as 1885 ozone was used in medical treatments. In Germany, ozone was used in many institutes until the second World War made an end to it. After the war the medical establishment forbade their members to use ozone, although several doctors were highly successful in treating patients with it.

Ozone, being a very concentrated form of oxygen, is a very powerful destroyer of bacteria, viruses and fungi. It also neutralizes pesticides, chemical wastes, poisons and odors. It is used widely in different industries. The home variety of ozone comes in pills, powders, potions and lotions, air purifiers, body suits, saunas and ozonated oils. As an example; when a car dealer wants to sell the car that belonged to a smoker, he will put an Ozon air purifier in the car. A day later you would not know that this was a smoker's car!

In health or in disease, do yourself a huge favor and buy Ed McCabe's book: *Flood Your Body With Oxygen.* It is a wealth of information which can save your life many times.

With the help of a physician, oxygen can even be given intravenously. To contact physicians who can assist you, visit this very informative website: *www.oxygentherapy.com* (doctors are listed by state).

When you have cancer and live close to a "Hyperbaric Center" (check your Yellow Pages) you may want to ask your doctor for a prescription for this treatment. Hyperbaric treatment consists of a two-hour stay in a large, oxygen-filled room where the atmospheric pressure is raised gradually. Because of the higher pressure, the blood will absorb more oxygen and will take it to oxygen-starved tissues, such as tumor-tissue, to bring healing. This same technique is also used in wound-healing. Ask your doctor if hyperbaric treatment is right for you! (I love to use that phrase, since it is being abused so often in commercials for drugs!)

Did you know that smart business people buy up, at a discount, sick cattle that are worn out from antibiotics and drugs; remove the drugs, ozonate the air and the water and then sell the cattle again a year later as healthy disease-free animals? (*Flood Your Body With Oxygen*; p. 227)

Oxygen and cancer cannot live together. Put the two together and oxygen will win, hands down.

Fight cancer and disease in general by loving up on oxygen and be educated in the many different and simple ways to boost your oxygen level.

Chapter 8

The Defense Factor

In Chapter 2 we mentioned that the absence of vitamin B_{17}, trypsin and progesterone is a requirement for cancer development, remember? We'll discuss the need for these substances in this chapter.

Before the second World War broke out in the Netherlands in 1940 many people were walking around sporting a little pin with a broken rifle. They believed in disarmament – if everybody puts down the arms and weapons the world will be a safer place. I'm sure many were sincere, but they were not right. Hitler's armies overwhelmed this little country and bombed the city of Rotterdam to smithereens in just two days.

Without the proper defenses our bodies too will easily succumb to the enemies of disease and sickness.

Three Weapons:

1. Trypsin. For a long time scientists pounded their heads against the wall because of the unexplainable fact that the body does not produce antibodies against cancer cells. *Why don't the white blood cells of the body's immune system take care of these cancerous* *cells*, they wondered. White blood cells travel around in the body as cops, arresting every substance or cell that is foreign, dead, or may bring damage to the body.

In 1905, professor of embryology at the University of Edinburgh, Scotland, John Beard came with the solution: cancer-cells have a protein coating with a negative electrical charge. White blood cells also have a negative charge and instead of being attracted to the cancer cells, they are repelled. That is why cancer cells aren't cleaned up by the white blood cells; they cannot come close to each other.

Thank God we were created with a back-up mechanism. The pancreatic enzyme, trypsin (and others), has been specifically designed to eat holes in the defensive protein coat of the cancer cell, after which the white blood cells can invade the cancer cell, kill it and gobble it up.

Way to go Trypsin!

2. Laetrile, or Vitamin B$_{17}$. In 1950 a scientist called Dr. Ernst T. Krebs, Jr. discovered a natural substance that very selectively kills cancer cells. He called it laetrile, also known by the name amygdalin. It has been regarded as a vitamin ever since – vitamin B$_{17}$. Laetrile works like a guided missile. Laboratory tests showed over and over again, in the presence of cancer cells, laetrile will selectively release a deadly load of cyanide, a very toxic substance, which destroys the cancer cells mercilessly on the spot without doing any harm to the healthy cells.

Isn't that a nice vitamin to have on board? Absolutely! It truly is a built-in gift from our creator to prevent cancer cells from needlessly developing into a tumor.

3. Progesterone. In Chapter 2 we briefly discussed the origin of the cancer process. Cancer is triggered when somewhere in our tissue there is a need for rapid cell-multiplication, for instance at a wound-site, but the multiplication is uncontrolled and "gets out of hand." We found that this was caused by a lack of cancer-*inhibitors*.

Let's talk about genes for a moment. When growth is taking place in a tissue of the body the command for cell-multiplication is given by a certain gene, let's call it the m-gene. Cell-death, on the other hand, is ordered by another gene, that we'll call the d-gene. The cancer-process is fired on by the activation of the m-gene and/or by de-activation of the d-gene. So, more m-gene commands more cells and more cancer. More d-gene commands less cells and lack of cancer.

Scientists have found that certain hormones play a crucial role in these processes. Estradiol, one of the hormones of the estrogen-group, turns on the m-gene and stimulates cell-multiplication (cancer). Progesterone, another hormone, turns on the d-gene that activates cell-death (anti-cancer). If both these hormones are available *in the proper concentration* there will be no cancer, because the cell will be able to regulate the processes in the right order. Progesterone opposes the estrogens and when both are in balance the replication process we call cancer will be kept in check.

So here they are: three weapons in the war against cancer:
- Trypsin
- Vitamin B_{17} (Laetrile)
- Progesterone

Our next question should be: with all this weaponry in our system, why do we still get cancer? And of course there is a very simple answer. *We have become deficient in these substances.* Our foods and food sources over the last fifty years have become so depleted of essential nutrients that in our age a regular diet does not provide us with the necessary ingredients for wellness. Our cells and immune systems lack these necessary weapons that form the right defense against cancer and so many other "modern" diseases. Cancer therefore can be regarded as a deficiency disease.

A call to rearm
- **Trypsin**, among other enzymes, is formed in the pancreas. Enzymes can be seen as substances that facilitate vital chemical formations in the body. Cancer patients do not produce enough of these enzymes either because, like diabetes patients, their pancreas is not functioning properly, or they are

already overwhelmed by cancer and the poorly working pancreas cannot keep up with the demand for trypsin.

An excellent supplement for pancreatic enzymes is **Wobenzym-N,** a German product that has proven itself in the past, having a wide range of enzymes, including trypsin. Check in Appendix C for where to purchase it. (One cause of a poorly performing pancreas can be a deficiency in vitamin C, so also read Appendix A.)

• **Laetrile**, or vitamin B_{17} deficiency is simply caused by our poor Western diet. B_{17} is found in the seeds of certain fruits and in vegetables; in apple seeds, for instance. When you chew an apple seed to pulp and taste the almond taste, you know that you found laetrile.

Have you ever been to the zoo and fed some fruits to the monkeys? What did you see? You saw the monkey run off with the fruit, peel the flesh of the fruit away and drop it, then crack the seed with his strong jaws and eat the soft inner part of the seed. After eating the kernel he would come back and eat the flesh of the fruit.

Laetrile works only together with the enzymes in the flesh of the apple, so always eat the seeds of the fruit *with* the flesh. Other foods that are rich in Vitamin B_{17} are alfalfa and other sprouts, apricot , cherry, peach and plum kernels, barley, beet tops, bitter almonds, blackberries, brewer's yeast, brown rice, buckwheat, cashews, cranberries, flaxseeds, garbanzo beans, lentils, lima beans, macadamia nuts, millet, pecans, raspberries, sorghum cane syrup, spinach, strawberries, walnuts, watercress and jams.

The apricot seeds contain the highest content of vitamin B_{17} on earth. As a preventative, Dr. Krebs asserts that seven to ten apricot seeds per day will make it impossible to develop cancer in one's life time. Wow, there's that good news again!

Vitamin B_{17} can also be purchased in the form of tablets for oral use and in vials, to be injected by a physician. One or two 100 mg tablets is a good maintenance dose to prevent cancer.

Now, before you run over to the drugstore, read on. Stores do not sell apricot seeds because of the raids the FDA made on those stores that sold vitamin B_{17} and apricot seeds years ago. It is extremely disappointing that the FDA has not yet given its approval to the therapeutic use of laetrile; a substance that is far less dangerous than a simple aspirin. This is why only a handful of physicians in the USA dare to use laetrile in their cancer treatment protocol. Isn't this a flagrant bullying of American citizens in favor of the pharmaceutical mafia?

It should be noted that, although laetrile is an excellent way to prevent and treat cancer, it may not have a therapeutic effect on brain tumors and basal cell carcinomas. Work with an alternative physician on this; he or she can guide you in the best approach to treat your particular condition.

And as said before, when one has cancer already, a more complicated protocol is required, including exercise, diet, enzymes and supplements. So find yourself a physician with enough guts and with an open mind to an alternative approach to fighting cancer. He or she will be able to help you. You will find addresses of doctors that want to help and of suppliers of laetrile in on the internet.

Highly recommended reading: *Laetrile Case Histories*, by John A. Richardson, M.D. and Patricia Irving Griffin, R.N., B.S. What a fantastic book; sixty-two case histories proving beyond any doubt that laetrile works in the control of cancer. This book also recounts the personal battle of Dr. John Richardson who incurred the wrath of the medical establishment when he and his patients elected to use vitamin therapy instead of surgery, drugs and radiation as treatment of choice.

• **Progesterone** deficiency is caused by two things: A lack of progesterone production in the body, or an imbalance. Progesterone is produced by the male as well as by the female body, although women make twice as much. After menopause or after hysterectomy (removal of the ovaries!) estrogen production decreases to 40%, but progesterone production is stopped completely, which creates a hormone imbalance. There is more estrogen than progesterone, or to put it in an other way, estrogens are not being opposed by the same amount of progesterone any longer. The result can be cancer, especially cancer of the uterus and breast cancer, which is the number one cancer in women.

Men only make half as much progesterone as women, but their testosterone works together with the progesterone to balance (oppose) the estrogens. After the age of forty-five most men's progesterone levels start to decrease. When this happens testosterone is converted into dihydrotestosterone which is useless in opposing the estrogens. Unopposed estrogen can then lead to cancer, specifically of the prostate, which is the highest ranking cancer in men.

The other cause of low progesterone can be a imbalance in the available amounts of progesterone and estradiol in the body. In our Western environment our bodies are flooded by an ocean of (petro-chemically manufactured) estrogens, like estradiol. You can find estrogens in cosmetic products, pesticides, meats, car exhausts, soap, furniture and carpeting fabrics and paneling, etc. We inhale, eat and drink all these different estrogens and when showering they are even being absorbed through the skin. Worst of all, after menopause, many women having hot flashes are still being put on (even more) estrogen by their physicians.

Because of this overabundance of estrogens the scales of the hormone balance are tipped heavily in favor of the estrogens. By the enormous availability of estrogens from the environment reaching our cells, the body's *normal* progesterone production can become inadequate and then estrogens like estradiol are not opposed any longer.

> We can conclude that women, after meno-pause, as well as men after forty-five have decreased levels of progesterone, which, according to many new studies, causes breast cancer in women and prostate cancer in men.

According to Dr. Joseph Mercola and Dr. John Lee, who was *the* international authority on hormone replacement therapy, "Breast cancer and prostate cancer both can be prevented and reversed by taking a small daily dose of natural progesterone cream."

Natural progesterone cream can be purchased at most health food stores. Progesterone is a fat-soluble substance which is best absorbed through the skin. So rub the cream on the inside of your arms or legs – wherever your skin is thinnest.

Dr. Lee prescribes his female patients to take a daily dose of 20 mg. Men can do with half this amount: 10 - 12 mg.

There are several companies that sell progesterone, but not all of them tell you the exact amount of progesterone in their product. Some producers have listened well to Dr. Lee and have put their product in a dispenser with a pump that gives a dab of exactly 20 mg. The dispenser for men gives exactly 10 mg.

Your local health food store may provide you with an audio tape of Dr. Lee, discussing the need for progesterone more in depth. We just heard that Dr. John Lee passed away. He was a champion for women's health issues.

Dr. Lee warned against the following:

> "Some physicians put women on Progestin and they tell their patients that this is exactly the same as progesterone. It is not! Progestin is a completely different molecule and is useless! Always make sure that your progesterone is real honest to goodness natural PROGESTERONE."

To summarize. In the fight against cancer, trypsin, vitamin B_{17} and progesterone have proven themselves to be important weapons in the prevention and reversal of cancer. All are being produced in the body, but the modern dietary challenges can leave us with drained and depleted systems, not being able to meet the growing demand.

Supplementing our systems with these natural substances is the most logical and health promoting thing to do. The products are safe, natural and welcome to the body. Just by taking any one of them *individually* people have been able to reverse their cancer.

Yes, you can win this battle! Keep on reading; there is much more!

Just before this book went to the printer I came across an English website that advertised a snack bar containing foods like apricot seeds that are known for their high amount of vitamin B_{17}, or laetrile.

The thought shot through my mind that it can be that easy to prevent cancer in America and far beyond. By daily eating a small candy bar filled with laetrile-containing foods we could prevent and eradicate cancer. If only we would let the researchers and the food industry run with it, cancer could be history!

Chapter 9

The Immunity Factor

*"Cancer is... a symptom of an
inefficient immune system."*
--A.E. Carter

The immune system is a network of specifically designed cells, communicating with the body to pick up signals of emergency, which trigger an immune response. The response can be compared to a police arrest. An emergency call is picked up, "dispatch" sends a message to a squad car that races to the place of emergency, the thief is surrounded and taken into the car, to be taken away from society.

In a similar way our God-given defense mechanism protects us against intruders and cleanses us from harmful body products. Needless to say, when our defense is down, sooner or later we will suffer the consequences. A poor immune system is a very important ingredient in the development of cancer.

In his book *The Cancer Answer*, A. E. Carter goes so far as to say that "Cancer is not a disease, but a symptom of an inefficient immune system." And further he adds: "Nothing causes cancer, but an inefficient immune system allows cancer to develop." His answer to cancer is: a healthy, active immune system!

Our immune system can be inadequate when the organs where the specific immune cells are formed, are diseased, which can happen as a result of, for example, radiation. Another reason for immunity failure can be the overburdening of a well functioning immune system.

In her book , *The Cure for All Diseases,* Dr. Hulda Clark tells us that the common cold is preceded by an overload of mold-toxins that kill, bind or gag the white blood cells of our immune system. While the white blood cells work at full capacity to take out the molds, the virus that causes the cold symptoms can then invade the cells of, for example, the lungs, and make us sick. So an invasion of toxic intruders can overload our immune system, which then is incapable of responding to normal duty.

The best time for robbing a bank is when there is a house on fire in the next block! There is only so much that one police unit can do!

For those who have been diagnosed with cancer (or any other chronic illness) it makes perfect sense to try to identify the reasons why your immune system did not defend you when cancer stuck up its ugly head.

So let's try to find what kept your immune system so busy. **Toxins** for example. Open a news magazine like *Time* or *Newsweek*, stick your nose in between the pages and smell; or rather, don't! What you'll smell are three to ten different carcinogens (toxins that cause cancer) from the paint, glue, paper, printing, etc. By the water we drink and bathe in, the air we breathe and the food we eat, all of us are daily exposed to a wide spectrum of toxic substances.

There is chlorine, pesticides, copper and fluor in our bath and drink water. On top of that, have a look at the labels and read all the unpronounceable names of petrochemical substances that are in our shampoos, soaps, body lotions, tooth paste and mouthwash, etc. The lists are endless.

Benzene, for example, a very toxic substance, was banned from all foods and cosmetics years ago. However it is showing up again in cosmetics, and traces of benzene are being found by Dr. Clark in all sorts of foodstuffs. The onslaught of toxins is really out of control in our Western culture. It will take a separate book to describe all these different toxins and types of pollution. *The Cure for All Diseases* by Dr. Clark tells in great detail how to find the source of toxins and how to deal with them.

Molds, fungi, viruses, parasites, etc. do not belong in your body. The reason they are there is that you are too toxic, and/or too acid! All the enemies mentioned above love the nice, warm environment that our body offers them. They are attracted to the many petrochemical substances in our tissues and to low pH tissue fluids. So get back to alkaline and don't show mercy to these critters, but kill all of them by using the zapper daily, and after you've become "clean", once a week for maintenance.

Free Radicals. Ever seen a pack of hyenas rip at a prey, like a buffalo? The buffalo out-sizes the hyena many times but the number of hyenas biting at the buffalo from every angle will eventually overpower the unfortunate animal. Often it is eaten alive while being held down from many different sides. It is a gruesome sight.

Free radicals are 'unhappy' molecules because they have one electron missing in their outer 'shell'. (An electron is a charged atomic particle) Their only aim in life is to become whole again. They will scavenge their environment for molecules that have an *easy to grab electron* and steel one if they get the opportunity. They are like the hyenas. Sometimes they find prey that is sick and dying and they will feast on the electrons from the dead cells in our tissues. This is their real function in life; they are part of the clean up crew in the body.

However when *too many* free radicals exist they will also start taking electrons away from *healthy* tissue. This can happen when your body has stored a high content of *'heavy metals'*, like lead, copper, iron, mercury, etc. Heavy metals are alien to the body. They do not belong there!

When a free radical bumps against a heavy metal molecule it results in a cascade of more, new free radicals.

Now you understand why it is so bad to store heavy metals in your body. Dental fillings and the metal used in piercings and tattoos will eventually leach their molecules into the bloodstream to be absorbed by the lining of the arteries triggering cardio vascular disease. Or these metals can end up in other tissues and cause free radicals to multiply and scavenge on healthy cells and even on genetic material in the cell nucleus, like the DNA. Some scientists believe the destruction of our DNA is at the origin of cancer.

When a free radical steels an electron from another molecule we call it *oxidation*. We say that the molecule that lost an electron was *oxidized*. Now, in order to keep free radicals from steeling, or oxidizing healthy cells and tissues, we need: *anti-oxidants*!

What are anti-oxidants? You guessed right; anti-oxidants are equipped with an <u>extra</u> electron to give away to the greedy radicals. Once the electron has 'jumped' from the anti-oxidant to the free radical, the radical stops being a radical and peace has returned to the tissues. Balance has been restored!

We could say that the tiny, electrically charged, electrons are the bringers and sustainers of life. *Electrons are life!* They are abundant in fresh fruits, vegetables and … blood. This is why animals that kill prey always first lap up the blood from the animal they killed. Blood is rich in electrons. God, however taught us, humans, not to eat blood but in stead to eat fruits and vegetables for their blood, or their …*juice*!

In a perfect situation you and I would only be eating fruits, nuts and vegetables. That was the original, God given diet. The free radicals in our tissues would only scavenge on the molecules from cells that were dying a natural death and because of the abundance of anti oxidants they would never touch healthy cells. This should be the normal situation.

We have talked much about the difference between alkaline and acid. An alkaline substance will always bring electrons into our body, while an acid substance will take electrons.

Well, since *too many* free radicals are such a problem and hazard to our health, we, first of all, need to find the outside source of free radicals and 'turn off the tap'. In our toxic environment they come as a multitude of different chemical substances. You'll find them in exhaust fumes, in printing dyes that we smell when we open a magazine, in the fabrics of furniture and car interiors, in paint, in air fresheners, in food preservatives, in the soaps and cosmetics we use, even in our food and drinks.

In our western lifestyle there is just no escape possible. So if we have to live with this daily stream of free radicals it is vital to also have a generous daily intake of anti oxidants!

It is helpful to know how many anti oxidants we can find in a food source, so in the next box you will find a list of *dried* fruits and vegetables with their ORAC value.

ORAC stands for Oxidant Radical Absorbance Capacity. It is a score for the anti oxidant potential of a fruit or vegetable. In a laboratory blood can be checked for its *'ORAC value'*. After eating for instance spinach, your blood will show a higher ORAC count.

Acai berry (freeze dried *'OptiAcai'*)	1027 (!)
Wild black Raspberry	340
Wild Blueberry	260
Elderberry	240
Spinach	150
Broccoli	130
Cranberry	95
Blueberry	93
Tomato	60
Blackberry	53
Carrot	50

So we need anti-oxidants, class!

As you've seen, the best source is fruits and vegetables.

When you are sick and you do not want to spend energy on chewing and digesting your food, the best way to get your anti oxidants, is by simply drinking fruit or vegetable juice. No need for chewing, no need for a whole lot of hydro-chloric acid in your stomach! Just pour in the goodness!

Following you will find a number of foods rich in anti oxidants, starting of course with:

☐ The **Acai berry**! As you see the Acai-berry (ah-sigh-ee) stands lonely at the top of the ORAC list. What a gem! So far I have found no better juice than MonaVie. MonaVie offers an impressive blend of 19 different fruits and berries with the Acai berry as the main ingredient. A special *'flash freeze'* patented procedure *(OptiAcai)* is used to maintain and *even increase* the anti oxidant power while processing the Acai berry.

Besides the anti oxidant power, the Acai berry is, simply put, a super food. It has the protein profile of eggs, it is high in fiber, it has essential fatty acids, natural vitamins and copious amounts of minerals and trace minerals. The Acai has a low glycemic index, so it is safe to take for diabetic people and it has cholesterol- and blood pressure lowering properties.

When you are battling with disease, what better food to take! In stead of bringing flowers you may want to give a bottle of this juice to a sick person. I personally have seen impressive results from people who have been drinking MonaVie.

A 26 year young guy I sat next to in a meeting showed me his face. He had a reddish spot on the right side of his face. He told me that this was the place where a tumor had been growing. *"When I started drinking MonaVie five weeks ago the tumor started shrinking and my pain is gone."* He drank 2 to 4 ounces every day. Needless to say that the guy was very excited and happy!

☐ **Krill oil** is another excellent natural source of anti oxidants. Krill are tiny shrimp-like crustaceans that live in the oceans. They are part of the plankton whales and other fish feed on. Only buy the purest form of Krill from the arctic oceans. (Always store your oil based supplements in the fridge!)

☐ **Microhydrin**. 1 - 2 Capsules 3 times per day, taken with plenty of water. (Every suggested dose is reckoned for adult bodies) Microhydrin is a new product manufactured by a genius inventor, Dr. Patrick Flanagan, who found a way to add one electron to every hydrogen atom. This may not strike you as much, but he claims that it is the most powerful anti-oxidant at the moment. One capsule of Microhydrin equals the anti-oxidant strength of 10,000 glasses of orange juice!! Microhydrin is sold as a food supplement and has been tried and tested by hundreds of medical doctors, with much reason for enthusiasm. It can only be purchased through certain websites or phone numbers.

☐ **Lycopene**. There is evidence that the lycopene in water-melon and tomatoes reduces the risks of certain types of cancer. It is a strong natural anti-oxidant.

☐ **Vitamin A**, 5000 IU's per day. (IU, or International Units) A healthy body converts beta-carotene from vegetables into vitamin A (called the immune vitamin!), however this does not seem to work for everybody. So be sure that you have enough, because Vitamin A is an important ingredient of the immune system. Too much Vitamin A can cause suppres- sion of bone building.

In a study from the University of Texas' M.D. Anderson Cancer Center 33% of leukemia patients treated with vitamin A were ...cured! They remained cancer free even after 5 years.

☐ **Vitamin E**, 400 - 800 IU's per day. Only buy the expensive kind! It will say: **d**-alpha Tocopherol, or gamma Tocopherol on the label. If the label reads **dl**-alpha Tocopherol it is made synthetically and, according to Dr. Len Horowitz and other health professionals, it is worthless.

Vitamin E consists of different substances, all called vitamin E. One of these: the Tocotrienols have shown to have an inhibiting effect on cancer and also on the growth of new bloodvessels that facilitates tumor growth. Hopefully science will be able to produce the Tocotrienols in a more concentrated form in the future.

☐ **Vitamin C**, 3000 - 5000 mg per day for maintenance. For therapeutic use of vitamin C in the treatment of cancer or other diseases I refer to Appendix B, which specifically deals with the therapeutic use of vitamin C.

☐ **Alpha Lipoic Acid** (ALA), 200 mg per day.

ALA neutralizes oil- based and water-based free radicals. It has demonstrated particular anti-oxidant protection of the heart and vascular system and it passes the blood brain barrier, so it reaches the brain.

Lester Packer, who heads a molecular and cell biology laboratory at the University of California at Berkeley, has shown that when vitamin E gives up an electron to that nasty free-radical, it then becomes a free-radical itself. But then vitamin C comes in to save the day, giving up one of its own electrons and thereby recycling the warrior power of E. He also has demonstrated that vitamin C (and vitamin E) is being regenerated by alpha lipoic acid, a powerful antioxidant, that the body produces itself in minute quan-tities. In fact, Packer believes lipoic acid is the most potent antioxidant of all and it's the only one known to easily get into the brain.

☐ **Selenium**, 200 mcg per day. This mineral is a strong anti-oxidant. It prevents cellular fats and lipids from going rancid and from producing aging spots and spots on the liver, amongst many other things.

☐ **Co-enzyme Q10**, 100 mg per day. Another strong anti-oxidant.

☐ **Zinc**, 50 mg per day. Vitamin A is dependent on this mineral to be able to be released from the liver into the bloodstream. Zinc strengthens and protects the Thymus, the immune system headquarters and is used in the production of anti-oxidant enzymes.

☐ **Germanium** -132, a trace mineral, 1 to 2 capsules of 150 mg on an empty stomach. The mineral Germanium has also been shown to promote healthy oxygen flow to tissues and normal functioning of immune-boosting cells!

☐ **Vanadium**, a metal, is active in causing the cancer cells to commit suicide (or apoptosis) within 4 to 24 hours. At this time research is on the way to develop Vanadium into a cancer-drug.

☐ **I3C** (Indole-3-carbinol) is a plant compound in some vegetables that has been proven to give anti-oxidant protection and to be effective against several types of cancer like colon-, lung-, breast-, and prostate-cancer. It inhibits cancer-cell growth and induces cancer-cell death. I3C is found in cabbage, radish and, you guessed right...Brussels sprouts. (Phoooj what a taste!)

Here is a little known Dutch secret: Brussels sprouts can only be 'enjoyed' when dipped in apple sauce. However, let's be thankful for scientists who can cram Brussels sprouts into tasteless capsules! As a vegetable extract I3C can be bought as a food supplement.

More good news: **cacao** (*not* mixed with milk) and **dark chocolate**, ladies, is very rich in anti oxidants and so is **green tea**.

Besides the free-radical chasers that are mentioned here there are many other ways to boost and strengthen the immune system.

Remember, it is better to be educated than to be medicated, so keep on reading and add some simple, natural lifesafers to the content of your kitchen cabinet.

☐ **Garlic.** Garlic seems to be the most effective anti cancer agent of the vegetables and the active ingredients have been identified. Take time to add some garlic to your cooking.

☐ **Taheebo**, also known as Lapacho Colorado and Pau D'Arco (Tabebuia impetiginosa), is a tree that is found in the rain forest near the Andes mountains in South America.

The inner bark of the tree is scraped and turned into a **tea**. As an immune-booster it has been used by the Indian people for centuries. It has an anti-tumor agent and possibly a large proportion of oxygen in solution. It has a pleasant taste.

☐ **Essiac Tea**, a harmless herbal tea, was used by Canadian nurse Renee Caisse (the name of the tea is the name Caisse spelled backward: Essiac!) to successfully treat thousands of cancer patients from the 1920s until her death in 1978 at the age of ninety. The Ontario nurse brought remissions to hundreds of documented cases, many abandoned as "hopeless" or "terminal" by orthodox medicine. The formula for the herbal remedy was given to Caisse in 1922 by a hospital patient whose breast cancer had been healed by an Ontario Indian.

Over the years, many prominent physicians voiced their support for the efficacy of Caisse's medicine. For example, Dr. Charles Brusch-a founder of the prestigious Brusch Medical Center in Cambridge, Massachusetts, testified, *"I endorse this therapy even today for I have in fact cured my own cancer, the original site of which was the lower bowels, through Essiac alone."*

☐ **Turmeric** is a herb that gives rice and curries their distinct yellow 'spicy' color. It can be used as a simple daily addition to many kinds of food and it is almost tasteless.

☐ The **Curcumin** in the Turmeric is a 'polyphenol that possesses not just one, but several anti cancer properties. Just look at all the benefits that this God given herb can give you: it is a strong anti-oxidant, according to University of Chicago scientists, Curcumin inhibits a cancer-provoking bacteria associated with gastric and colon cancer, Curcumin blocks estrogen and estogen-mimicking chemicals that promote cell mutation and growth. These chemicals are found everywhere in our industrialized environment.

Curcumin inhibits cyclo-oxygenase (COX) and lipoxygenase (LOX), two enzymes that promote inflammation believed to play a significant role in the development and progression of colon cancer, it inhibits angiogenesis, or the process by which tumors create their own blood supply, it destroys abnormal pre-cancer cells and stops cancer cells from multiplying and it enhances the immune system.

Indian researchers have mentioned that Curcumin may be a very safe alternative to chemo treatment and they are trying to prove this.

☐ In the sixties a mushroom called **Agaricus blazei Murill** became famous for its incredible immune boosting properties. In Piedade, Brazil, people were noticed for their extraordinary health by eating their favorite mushroom *'Cogumelo do Sol'*. Japanese scientists studied the mushroom for its medical properties and found it had anti tumor properties in guinea pigs. Cancerous guinea pigs experienced a recovery rate of *99 percent* when they were treated!

This mushroom contains a list of components that stimulate the immune system by activating T-cells, macrophages, Interleukin and tumor necrosis factors.

☐ **Graviola** (Annona Muricata)

You may have heard about Graviola. Graviola products (capsules and tincture) have become more available on the American market place. The acetogenins in the Graviola leaves, bark, fruits and seeds have been subject of research for quite a while and they have been found to have a strong toxic effect on many different cancer cells, especially those cells that are resistant to other therapy.

It gets even better because Graviola products are also very selective in killing *only* cancer cells and that gives Graviola a wonderfull edge in relation to the extremely harsh chemo-treatment that so severely weakens the *whole* physical (immune) system.

The therapuetic dosage of graviola leaf is reported to be 2-3 grams taken 3 or 4 times per day. A wonderful, God given, natural and safe product to use in your fight against cancer.

One of the action mechanisms of Graviola is the depletion of ATP (energy) to cancer cells. The main supplement that increases ATP is Coenzyme Q10, mentioned earlier as a strong anti-oxidant.

So when taking Graviola you may want to hold off on the Co Q10 for a while.

☐ **Sauerkraut** has been found to have cancer fighting pro-perties that encourage precancerous cells in the digestive system to self-destruct, a process known as apoptosis.

☐ In an article from Reuter's Health News, Dr. Jennifer Rhode stated: "In multiple ovearian cancer cell lines we found that **ginger** induced cell death at a similar or better rate that the platinum-based chemotherapy drugs typically used to treat ovarian cancer."

In the same article it was said that **Capsaicin**, which makes chili peppers so hot, causes cell death, but does not effect healthy cells

☐ The University of South Carolina did a studie with **Ellagic acid**, derived from fruits like raspberries, on 500 patients with cervical cancer. Nine years later they could conclude that Ellagic acid inhibits and stops cancer-cell division in 48 hours and causes normal cell death (apoptosis) in 72 hours. Different products are on the market, make sure to read the labels and see how much of Ellagic acid is actually in a capsule! There is fraud going on also in the vitamin world, so check and see if your daily serving is closest to 840 mg (6 caps).

☐ **Noni juice, XanGo** and **Mangosteen** are juices harvested from exotic tropical fruits with healing properties that have been known for thousands of years. Fruits and berries are the best a tree or shrub has to offer. The seeds that carry the genetic material for a new brush or tree have to make a good start. Just like we give to our children the best of the best, nature gives its best gifts to posterity in the form of a fruit or a berry.

There are many stories of people having used just these juices in the healing of their cancer and other diseases and of doctors prescribing it to their patients. They are still pretty expensive but folks, it's worth the money!

Every half hour take a little zip of the juice in your mouth and just swish it around so the juice can be absorbed straight into the bloodstream without having to go through the stomach and digestive tract.

☐ Several large studies recently concluded the effective-ness of **coffee** and even **tea** in preventing a number of different types of cancer. A daily cup of 'wake-me-up', real cafeinated coffee reduces the risk of breast cancer among pre menopausal women an impressive 40% and also cuts considerably in the risk of colon and liver cancer. The use of decafeinated coffee did not show anything worth writing about.

Chances of getting ovarian cancer can be cut down by 46% when drinking 2 cups of green or black tea per day. Women who only drank 1 cup still reduced their risk by 24%.

Any cup over and above the 2 per day showed even better numbers; every cup gave an *18% increased reduction*! That, dear ladies, is VERY good!

Put that on your 'Tea'- shirt and wear it!

And yes, I hear you, male ones! You men would like to know if coffee and tea will also keep *your* ovaries from cancer?

Sure! Male ovaries are called testes, guys. During the period of gestation ovaries and testes spring from the same 'sprung', so it will be very likely that men find the same kind of protection from their cup of 'pick-me-up'.

Do not forget, however, that coffee and tea dehydrates the body, so also drink plenty of water.

☐ **Glyconutrients.** (Glyco = sweet)

I can fill a whole chapter just about these sugary nutrients. No, I am not about to tell you to add sugar to your diet; at least not the kind of sugar you sprinkle over donuts. The sugars we're talking about here are 'essential' sugars, the stuff we absolutely cannot live without.

The very recent discoveries made by the scientists studying these 'essential sugars' take place on one of the last frontiers of bio-chemistry.

I will let an insider do the talking here.

Dr. Iain McRobert has written an open letter to inform us about this new and very promising approach to health.

"An open letter to mank;nd

In the last twenty years, a huge and grow;ng body of research has been carr;ed out ;nto the role of the sugars that are an essent;a/ part of glycoprote;ns. These sugar-prote;n complexes are the bui/d;ng blocks of our ;mmune system, and are the method by wNch cells "talk" to each other. Research now runs to over 80,000 papers ;n many estabHshed med;cal journals. The accompany;ng papers ;n this pack discuss various aspects of sugar metabolism, tram the sdent;t;c research to case histories, along w;th doctors own exper;ence w;th the amazing heaHng qua/Wes of these glyconutr;ents.

(Note: There are over 200 sugars found in nature - only 8 have been deemed "essent;a/" - the common table sugar is one we all get way too much of in our diet and is NOT one of the sugars that is deemed "essential".)

It has been conclusively shown that there are 8 essential sugars (out of the 200), and 6 are missing tram our modern Western d;et. This lack is caused by soil depletion, early p;cking of vegetables and truits, processing of foods, and pollution. We all now face a very toxic environment, and we now lack the very things we need to cope with the toxic load.

"When these "essential' sugars are m1ss1ng, the cells either cannot "talk," or they miscommunicate. The result is disease. Yes it is true, our cells can make these sugars 'from glucose, but this is a very metabolically expensive process. It has been shown that dietary lack results in defective immune response, either too much or too little. Allergic conditions are examples of an over reactive immune system. An under reactive immune system could result in an inability of the natural "killer" cells (lymphocytes) to recognize diseased or cancerous cells, and dispose of them. The results of that may mean the death of the person! When the cells are given the nutrients they need, and begin to function properly, the resultant health benefits range from profound to amazing. In some cases, the so called laws of medical science have been overturned. I have spoken to people who had (past tense) multiple sclerosis, and who now do not have it. Their neurological lesions have disappeared from the MRI scan. To a natural skeptic like myself, the implication of this reversal was simple - medicine is now facing the need for a total paradigm shift in its thinking, as deep a shift as that which occurred when bacteria were first shown to be the agents of infectious diseases.

As doctors, I believe we need to move from a "curative" view to a "wellness" view of what we do. Whilst modern medicine has made great strides in many areas, doctors, myself included, feel somewhat helpless when attempting to deal with the flood of degenerative disease and chronic illness that are the mark of our generation. All we can offer are drugs with very serious, and in some cases, life threatening side effects. In the year 2000, more than 7 00,000 people died from the effects of properly prescribed, properly administered pharmaceutical agents in the United States alone. This does not count the tragic accidents of improperly used medication.

Are these sugars safe? Well, they are food, not drugs. They have NO toxic or side effects. Five of the eight are found in human breast milk, (one of the reasons why babies are protected from disease by breast feeding). The sugars are not pharmaceutical agents, and do not cure anything. They simply restore basic cellular functions to normal, and then the body can fend for itself The killer cells will work to identify and destroy diseased or cancerous cells. The immune system can be restored to normal to modulate itself in response to attack.

I believe that we are going to see this profound change in medical practice over the next few years. As usual, I predict that the medical profession will be dragged kicking and screaming into this change. Every major medical advance, from simple hand washing between patients, to using limes to treat scurvy, to smallpox vaccination, the introduction of anesthesia, and surgical asepsis, has been first ridiculed, then opposed, until finally acceptance came when the truth became totally self evident.

This is happening today with glyconutrition. There are now over 7000 medical practitioners in the USA who regularly use glyconutrients in their practices. The AMA in Australia has just release a paper acknowledging the patient's right to use complimentary medicine. That statement allows such things as acupuncture and yoga, techniques that may have benefit, but have no scientific validation. Compare that to the huge body of literature on glycoscience, including the 7 999 Nobel Prize in Medicine.

The case history data is growing into the tens of thousands of patients whose disease states have been improved, or in many cases eradicated, by the simple act of adding these sugars to the diet. This evidence will, in time, be overwhelming, and those who are skeptical and critical will be won over, by evidence that cannot be refuted. When you have CAT scan evidence of the lesions of multiple sclerosis disappearing, of metastatic carcinoma resolving, of the reversal of Alzheimer's and Parkinson's disease, of increase in IQ of Down's syndrome children, along with positive effects in arthritis, infections, chronic fatigue syndrome, fibro-myalgia, what can you say? These are case histories presented by medical professionals, not snake oil salesmen. They are medically verifiable.

I think you will find the accompanying papers interesting. I hope that they will increase your understanding, and help you on the road to optimal health. Further information can be had at: www.glycoscience.org.

We started this chapter with the idea that cancer is a symptom of a failing immune system. After reading these pages I trust you found enough 'items' to work on.

When you are treated for a disease by a physician and take medications, please realize that some of these medications are very sensitive to any sudden change in diet. Always first inform your doctor if you plan to change to a more healthy diet so he or she can monitor you and fine-tune your medication. Coumadin, or Warfarin, for instance, are drugs that thin the blood, but so do other substances in vegetables and fruits. One of my neighbors who is on Coumadin found that out when he ate twice as much salad on a Saturday and punctured his skin while working in the yard. The bleeding almost could not be stopped. Isn't this a curious treatment? This Coumadin interferes with natural blood thinners, so we are not to change to a more healthy diet as long as we use it...!?? Do I smell a rat?

Chapter 10

The Ignition Factor: a Shocking Truth

This chapter will cover the last of the seven factors or prerequisites for tumor growth that we have discussed in Chapter 2. Here we'll discuss one factor that triggers the cancer process in such an unexpected way that I deliberately put it at the end of this group of chapters.

For some of you the subject dealt with here would very well take you completely by surprise and cause you to throw the book in a corner. I don't want you to start off thinking that cancer "is all in your head," because it's not!

We have talked a lot about the conditions that will set the stage for and will promote cancer, but the question remains: What really is it that starts cancer or tumor growth? Well, if there would be a clear answer, we all would know it by now.

Let's be a bit more precise. If all the conditions and "ingredients" for tumor growth have come together:

- the environment of the cells is acid and deprived of oxygen,

- our cell defense is down, and parasites are up,
- our WMD's are missing,
- our cell walls have deteriorated,

If all these cancer facilitators are set in place, what is it then that triggers normal cells to start behaving like tumor cells?

So far there is no conclusive answer. Many scientists will point to the nucleus of the cell, where the genetic material of the cell is stored and where the DNA signals its commands to the tiny cell organs, like the mitochondrions that function like little energy generators. There, somewhere at the microscopic level, the trigger for cancer must take place, they say. Probably, by cosmic radiation coming from space or by man-made radiation like X-rays, the cell nucleus is damaged, genetic material is "mutated," causing the DNA to send a wrong message, resulting in abnormal function of the cell organs, which may start the tumor process.

The other answer that I've found is given by Dr. R. G. Hamer, a German doctor who headed up a cancer clinic, fell ill with cancer himself and survived. He says he can locate the onset of a tumor growth at an exact moment in time. Here is how he came to his fascinating conclusions.

In 1987 his son, Dirk Hamer, who had been shot in a freak accident, died in his arms after a four-month struggle for his life. Shortly after, Dr. Hamer contracted testicular cancer. He had a suspicion that the death of his son had to do with his own condition and he started to investigate this possibility. Being a doctor in a cancer clinic gave him the opportunity to compare enormous amounts of cancer case histories. He found that every cancer had started with a trauma, a shock, an event experienced like a sudden stroke of lightning, something that "hits" you out of the blue and catches you completely unprepared – an event that rocks you on your foundations. People who had this happen will tell you their hands turned cold as ice, their hearts stopped beating for a moment, their breathing caught, their appetite left them, they could not sleep for days and had their minds completely occupied by the traumatic event.

For instance, the sudden death of a loved one, a sudden fear for loss of life during an airplane emergency, or a very bad diagnosis from a doctor that totally catches one by surprise. (Dr. Hamer called such a trauma a DHS, or a Dirk Hamer Syndrome, after the shock of the death of his son Dirk Hamer.)

You may think now: "Oh, yeah, it's the old mind over matter argument." But wait! I have a strong argument to give Dr. Hamer more credit. Dr. Hamer has very solid proof! When the brains are scanned after a DHS, a clear, target like mark (circles inside a circle) appears on the cat-scan of the brain, which is easy to see even with an untrained eye. Even the director of the Siemens Corporation that produces the cat-scan equipment has confirmed Dr. Hamer's findings.

The location of the target mark on the brain is determined by the type of conflict that was experienced. A loss, an injury, a fear, all these have their own location on the brain, and since our brain is in direct contact with all the tissues and organs in our body, the location of the target mark on the brain determines where the tumor will manifest itself. For example, when the DHS is a sudden fear of death, like during a plane crash, it will leave a target mark on the brain- stem, which has nerve connections with the lung. So, a sudden fear of death can trigger cancer in the lung.

> *Once more:* A sudden traumatic event that hits us like a bolt of lightning can be experienced by us as a DHS. The trauma causes swelling in a specific area in the brain, showing up on a cat-scan as a target mark. The place on the brain is determined by the *kind* of trauma. The change in brain tissue somehow causes tumor growth in a specific tissue or organ. Not every traumatic event is experienced by us as a DHS; consequently not every trauma will ignite tumor growth.

Dr. Hamer's ideas about health have been proven and can all be verified, contrary to conventional cancer treatment that is based mostly on theory and statistics. Yes, you can prove almost anything with statistics!

He has assisted many cancer patients back to health and has given us a new, more holistic approach to disease and sickness. He calls his approach to medicine: the "Germanic New Medicine," where he makes a very convincing case for the mind-body connection in healthcare.

As this chapter was written, Dr. Hamer, who is 70 years old, is locked up in a jail in France. Since he did not practice *'consensus medicine'* (only doing what all other doctors do), his doctor's license was taken from him, which made him an outlaw trying to cure people from cancer. He was not allowed to lecture on his "New Medicine" at a convention held in Spain. Here we see how far the medical (cancer) mafia can spread its tentacles even on an international level.

Not every one who lives through a DHS contracts cancer. Since a low pH (high acidity) is a very strong factor for cancer, perhaps only the *combination* of a DHS and a high acidity will produce tumor growth. It would be a great subject for further research.

How can you benefit from Dr. Hamer's approach in the here and now of *your* situation? If we may believe Dr. Hamer, the cancer process is ignited right after a sudden trauma that leaves a mark on the brain. The connection between the brain and the tissues where the cancer is triggered is bridged by the nervous system – nerve fibers that reach from the brain to every part of the body. That would mean that our own brain could be responsible for triggering the tumor process in our tissues. It gives a lot of food for thought and for further research.

The nature of traumas is such that we cannot avoid them; otherwise we would not call them traumas. They happen to each and every one of us. Most traumas do not hit us like a DHS, however sometimes they do and then they can ignite, or trigger cancer.

The good news is that, according to Dr. Hamer, the healing phase of cancer starts when the psychological conflict has been dealt with. When we've come to grips with our sudden fear or loss; when we've digested our psychological trauma, then the tumor growing phase is halted and the target mark on the brain-scan can be seen to fade away. Perhaps it is the sudden overload in the emotional part of the brain that causes the target formation on the other brain components. It is important then, from a *prevention* point of view, that we do not allow psychological traumas to linger on in our minds. The sooner we consciously deal with the emotions that came with the trauma the quicker the healing phase sets in. If you are battling with cancer right now, you'll want to eradicate any trauma that left you emotionally "paralyzed" or startled.

Close this book for a moment and go back in time. Check your mind and your emotions and see if anything comes up that may have caused a DHS. And if there is, then here's what to do:

- Talk about it with a friend, a counselor, a partner, or some one you trust. Take the time to express your feelings about the event ...from the bottom of your heart!

- Overcome the hurt, the fear, the mental pain, the anguish, or anxiety that was felt at the time of the trauma. Grieving, sadness and mourning is good …for a period of time. It should not continue on for months and months.
- Pray about it …from the bottom of your heart!
- If you need to: forgive your neighbor or yourself from the bottom of your heart!

Sometimes, after you've done all the right things, the memories, the fear, or the anxiety, or just your "nerves" still keep you awake and hold you in a grip that does not want to let go. They just keep going around and around in your nervous system and manifest in cold sweats, persistent thoughts, tremors, shortness of breath, a feeling of being choked, irregular heartbeats, neck or back pain, nightmares, raised blood pressure, phobias, etc.

There is a solution to all of that! In Appendix A you will find a surprisingly effective technique that comes close to an acupuncture treatment. You can do it all by yourself. It is simple to memorize and to practice it and it is very effective in getting the control back over your mind and body. Please do not skip this appendix!

You have now learned what it is that may have ignited your tumor and what to do about it. To prevent any new cancer from igniting I give you some more food for thought in the following:

Do not put yourself or your loved ones in harm's way and stay away from situations where you know you may "get the scare of your life," or "freak out." Let me name a few situations and places: hurricanes, movie cinemas, home videos, roller coasters, hospitals, some tv programs, etc. Do not underestimate the effect of a movie on your emotional brain. Remember *The Exorcist?* Many people have been and still are severely traumatized by it!

Dr. Hamer has found that many different cancers are being needlessly ignited through the fear that is often triggered by doctors giving their patients a somber diagnosis. Could this be the trigger of new tumor growth we call metastasis?

This chapter is being written at the time we see the horror taking place in New Orleans after it was smashed by Hurricane Katrina. People are losing everything they have and are scared of their lives being taken in a city submerged by water, darkness, looting and anarchy.

When I had my son read this chapter to see if my message came across, he said to me: "Dad, there are going to be many cancer victims in the New Orleans area in the coming months and years..." I think he got the message.

Please read more about Dr. Hamer's approach in my new book: **"The Cause and Cure of Breast Cancer"**. A must for any (young) woman having to deal with breast cancer. When you know the cause of cancer, you can prevent it and, or fight it successfully. More in the end of this book.

Information about Dr. Hamer, on the following website: WWW.Learninggnm.com.

Chapter 11

The Forgotten Vitamin: H2O!

Chapter 11 is about water, perhaps *the* most important nutrient for our body.

When we have to fight cancer, the consumption of clean, pure, electrically charged, clustered water may very well be the most vital thing you can do to improve your health.

Doctor Lorraine Day, MD, in her info-video "Cancer Does Not Scare Me Anymore," tells the story of her own fight with breast cancer. On her web-site she even showed a picture of the tumor on her breast. One of her weapons was: drinking many glasses of pure water every day. She survived!

We are not drinking enough water. Especially when people get older they tend to substitute coffee, tea, diet sodas, and even alcoholic beverages for water simply because of the nice taste. Many don't realize that all fluids are not created equal.

Dr. F. Batmanghelidj, MD, warns us to "Avoid drinks with caffeine or alcohol as they can dehydrate you." Why?

> Every six ounce drink with caffeine or alcohol requires an additional 10 to 12 oz. of water to re-hydrate your body!

When you have been a notorious coffee drinker for years, you can only imagine how much your whole system has suffered under dehydration. In his book, *Your Body's Many Cries For Water* Dr. Batman advises to use "The Water Cure Recipe," which goes as follows:

Drink 1/2 your body weight of water in ounces, daily. Example 180 lb. = 90 oz. of water daily. Divide that into 8 or 10 oz. glasses and that's how many glasses you will need to drink, daily. Use 1/4 teaspoon of salt (non-refined ocean- or sea salt) for every quart of water you drink. As long as you drink the water and it isn't prohibited by your physician, you should be able to add the salt.

Many people also suggest starting the day with up to five or six glasses of water and then waiting at least an hour before eating or drinking anything. Be sure to start out slowly and build up to this. You can overdo this if you try to drink too much too quickly while your body isn't used to it. (Some call this drowning.)

There are many reasons why drinking much water is essential to good health. Water consists of two vital elements: oxygen and hydrogen. Without either of them, we cannot live.

Pure water has a pH of 7.0. When you have found yourself to be too acidic, drinking pure water is another way of alkalizing your system back to normal values. Really pure alkaline water, however, is extremely hard to find, so we need to talk about this a little more.

All people groups that enjoy longevity and remarkable health have been found to have one thing in common: clean, toxin-free, mineral rich, electrically charged, clustered water. Most of them live high in the mountains and obtain their water straight from little streams that originate from the glaciers. Glaciers slowly slide down the mountains and grind and pulverize the rock that is trapped at the bottom. This rock-powder dissolves into the water and reaches the little streams that feed the rivers. The water of these rivers has a milky color because of the very high content of minerals. Groups like the Hunza people drink their water straight from these little rivers and they irrigate their fields with it, which results in lush growing fruits and vegetables with a high mineral content.

Tap-water has been fluoridated, radiated, chlorinated and who knows what else they've done with it. Both fluoride and chlorine are very toxic to our physical systems.

Well-water can contain pesticides, toxins and too much of a particular kind of a mineral, like iron.

Natural spring-water, the kind you buy in plastic bottles in the supermarket, may be good, but it also may contain a wrong mineral content, or it can pick up petroleum substances like benzene, that is used in the cleaning of the bottling machines. Dr. Hulda Clark found traces of benzene, an extreme toxic substance, in almost every kind of spring-water with her very sensitive equipment.

Distilled-water may be a better option; however, all the important minerals that are supposed to be in our drinking water have been distilled out of this type of water. Distilled water is also expensive and may have traces of benzene.

You see, it isn't easy to find something as simple as plain, clean and pure water.

Many respectable health guru's choose water that has been filtered by a system called **reverse osmosis.** A membrane filters out 99.9% of anything that is in the water: toxins, sediment, minerals, etc. So, although the water is cleansed and safe to drink, it has also lost nearly all of its minerals, like calcium, magnesium, etc. We must replenish them! A reverse osmosis unit can be bought at most do-it-yourself stores for around $150 – and it fits under the sink.

Another, cheaper option is a carbon filter. These come in a wide variety and will fit on the sink, next to the tap, or on the tap. Carbon filters eliminate the poisonous chlorine and the sediment, but leave many of the minerals and pesticides in the water.

And if you do not have a filter at all, you can take your water from the tab and just let it stand for a couple of hours. The chlorine will evaporate from the water, so at least you have taken out the worst poison.

Whichever way you choose to filter the water, keep in mind that you'll have to replenish your body with the important minerals and trace-minerals that were taken out, in order to keep your body alkaline.

(Don't drink your water from soft plastic bottles. When above room temperature the plastic leaches toxins into the water which accumulate in your tissues. I found hard plastic bottles, made from poli-carbonated plastic that does not leach its toxins into the water!)

• • •

As mentioned before, Hunza-water has an electrical charge. It is rich in electrons and has subsequently a high pH of more than 8.0; it is *very* alkaline.

It is interesting to test the water that you drink at home, with your Litmus paper. I found that my tap-water has a pH of 5.0 and my reverse-osmosis water also had a disappointing pH of not more than 5.0. My well water did a little better: 5.5. So, although my family and I drink reverse osmosis water, there is not much life (free electrons) left in it.

To super-charge and super-alkalize your dead drinking water, you can take half of a capsule of **microhydrin powder** (break open a capsule or buy the powder) and add it to a glass of water. Immediately it will charge your water from a poor pH of 5.0 to a pH higher than 8.0.

Microhydrin also detoxifies the chlorine in tap water; it brings the surface tension of water to where the cells of the body like it to be and lastly it will make the water form clusters, or chain linked water molecules, that make it easier for the cells of the body to absorb water.

Alternately, buy a bottle of **hydracel**. It is made from the same substance as microhydrin, and it will do the same thing for your drinking water. Since hydracel is a very concentrated liquid, it comes in a small bottle; small enough to put into a lady's purse to be available wherever you are. Whether it is at home, in the car or in a restaurant, now you can drink "living water" all through the day and bring your system back to alkaline. Just add several drops to your drink and voila!

Finally, in the chapter on "Stinkin' Thinkin'" we discussed the work of Mr. Emoto, who shows in his pictures of water crystals that love and gratitude have a definite impact on the formation and the "character" of water.

In our good ol' U.S. of A., we take the water that flows out of our tap and showerhead for granted. In Africa, where mothers have to get their often dirty water from miles away and have to carry it in tanks on their head, I have seen water treated like it was a favorite pet. At these places water is life and the lack of it means death.

Let's speak out with gratitude to our creator for the endless stream of life that we have such easy access to. It serves Him right and it may even revitalize the water we give daily to our God-given bodies. *L' chaim! ...to life!*

Chapter 12
Dos and Don'ts

Here are some more general guidelines for good health, gleaned from a wide range of doctors and authors.

Detoxify your body! In the course of a lifetime toxins will accumulate in the body. Your liver is the main cleaner-upper, however, if your liver has been clogged up for many years the toxic substances are not filtered out of your body but stored away in your tissue. For example, mercury. If you ever had amalgam put into your teeth by the dentist, you will be contaminated with mercury. Again, Dr. Hulda Clark's book: *The Cure for all Diseases* is probably the best source. She makes detoxifying sound simple and gives you many ways to cleanse your body, your house and garage of all the bad stuff. A must-read!

Regularly **cleanse your liver and kidneys**. They are the filters of your circulation. Ever changed the air filters of your air conditioning after two years? Then you know what that mess looks like. As you progress in age your body filters need to be cleansed as well. It is a very easy job. Again, find out what your health shop has in store for you. The kidneys are often cleansed by drinking a tea drawn from special herbs. Dr. H. Clark's liver cleanse is fast and very effective. You're done in one day and the results are absolutely remarkable. You will find cholesterol that has clogged up the ducts in your liver in little balls floating in the toilet bowl after you're done and your energy level will shoot up. (From: *The Cure for all diseases*, by Hulda Clark.)

As said before, do not eat **hydrogenated fats**, or anything that contains **trans-fatty acids**. It's very bad for your cell walls. Watch the labels! (Mayonnaise, margarine, vegetable oils, corn oil, etc.) Cold pressed olive oil is a good oil, but do not heat it. Only coconut oil is safe to use when frying. Make your own spreads and mayonnaise with the right kind of oils. Eat butter instead of margarine! Even your dog and cat won't eat margarine! Margarine is not a food!

The fat in **homogenized milk** has been artificially altered and scientists have spoken out their concern that homogenized milk can be a major cause of heart disease. So drink un-homogenized raw milk instead. Cow milk is too high in protein content; drink goat milk instead. It is more like human (mother's) milk.

Coffee, tea, and soda-drinks not only acidify, but also **dehydrate** your body; so when you drink any of them it forces more water out of your cells than it will bring in, eventually damaging your cells.

Use the food chart in Chapter 5 to pick your groceries. Always try to eat more **alkalizing foods** than acid foods; eat seventy-five percent alkalizing foods and twenty-five percent acidifying foods. If you had too much meat one day, eat a fruit salad for lunch and dinner the next day to get yourself back in balance.

One of the best ways to get well fast is to buy a 'juicer' for approximately $200. (Buy a "slow rotating" juicer, so the juices are not overheated.)

Carrots have beta carotene, an important anti-oxidant (Anti-oxidants help our bodies fight free radicals). When you eat one carrot it takes you a few minutes to chew it all into little bits and pieces. After you swallow it your stomach will separate the juice from the pulp. The pulp goes down south and out the far end, but in your intestinal tract the juice is absorbed into your blood and will eventually reach the cells. Notice that only the juice will reach your cells. Now take a juicer and juice ten carrots. In three minutes you'll have a whole glass of carrot juice that, when you drink it, *will go straight to your cells.* No need for digestion, you save the precious alkaline digesting juices for when you really need them. With a juicer you can prepare raw, uncooked food that is immediately available for your cells. Can you imagine how tickled your cells will be? It is also a great way to lose weight. Since your cells will not tell your brain any longer that they are in constant need of cell-food, your hunger pains will disappear.

Do not eat old bread or spoiled fruit. The molds that they carry can overwhelm your immune system, so that other, opportunistic diseases, like the cold or flu-virus can take their chance and make you sick.

When you have been diagnosed with cancer, try to stay away from any **refined sugars**, since they are fueling the cancer-cells.

According to the front-page article in the *Reader's Digest* of August 2003, "How Safe Is Your Food?" we need to think twice before we have another tuna, shark, or swordfish steak. The big predators of the ocean, but also fresh-water fish, like bass and trout have been found to be contami-nated with **mercury,** one of the worst toxins on earth. So be careful as to what kind of fish you have for dinner.

Mercury is used also in the amalgam the dentist fills your cavities with. You'd think that by now the whole medical (dental) world would have abandoned any application where mercury is involved.

Where is the FDA in this matter? Talk with your dentist and never let him put amalgam in your teeth. As a matter of fact, you would do good to have the amalgam in your mouth removed by a knowledgeable dentist. It has to be taken out with the utmost care so that no spilled particles of it can end up in your digestive tract, where it can continue to poison you. *Take responsibility for your health!*

Chewing gum. Chewing gum releases **mercury** from the amalgam fillings in your teeth. Now the mercury can end up in any part of your body! Chewing also stimulates the secretion of digestive enzymes in your pancreas and acid in your stomach to help you digest. When you chew gum you are needlessly causing the stimulation of these digestive processes, loosing precious alkalinity and irritating the lining of your stomach.

Do not drink water from soft **plastic bottles** or jugs. When the plastic heats up above room temperature or is frozen (in the delivery truck), toxins (organo-chlorines) will leach from the plastic into the water and will reduce the pH of the water. These organo-chlorines were found in the breast tissue of women with breast cancer! I recently found *policarbonate* plastic bottles in the health food store. The plastic from these bottles does not leach its toxins into your drinking water

Cell phones and cordless **phones** generate a pretty strong electro-magnetic energy field. This energy force does not stop at your skin or your skull; it literally messes with your brain. The British Health Protection Agency has admitted an increased association between acoustic neuromas, a type of ear tumor that can cause deafness, and the electromagnetic fields emitted by these telephones. A study has shown that the risk of cordless phone users developing these neuromas has doubled over the course of a decade.

The strong transmitter of the cordless phone is found in the part that holds the charger and the answering machine. Do not place this close to your bed or favorite chair!

When you hold your cell phone close to the car radio when it is transmitting, the radio and even your TV start squeaking. The same interference happens inside your brain and other tissues when you hold the phone close to your ear or when you're close to the charging unit!

For the same reason: do not get too close to anything that transmits energy, like computers, microwaves, tv-sets, electric heaters, and – I'm sorry to say, electric blankets. All these will put your health at risk, but the next one is a real killer.

Medical X-rays. Two studies by John Gofman, M.D., Ph.D., Professor Emeritus, Molecular and Cell Biology, (in 1996 and in 1999) *both* found that in the United States, ionizing radiation from medical x-rays is a necessary co-factor causing breast-cancer (between seventy-five and ninety percent of the cases). The 1999 study finds that medical x-rays are a necessary co-factor in over fifty percent of all other types of cancer, and sixty percent of coronary artery disease. Press releases about the studies, issued by the University of California, have been ignored by the media.

In plain English: x-rays are not safe! Ask your doctor to minimize this type of examination as much as possible and when you have to have x-rays taken, for instance with a mammogram, double up on your intake of anti-oxidants like Vitamin C and E before and after treatment.

Better yet, ask your doc for **thermography** instead of x-rays. Thermography is a technique where a heat detection screen is used to find hotspots in the breast tissue. Hotspots appear when more blood is flowing to a cancerous part of the tissue. No radiation! It is safe and it can even find a cancer two to three years earlier than a regular mammography.

Now that we talk about **breasts**, we need to talk about the bra (short for brassiere). Sydney Ross Singer and Soma Grismaijer, found in a study involving 4,700 U.S. women, that women who wear a bra twenty-four hours a day had a cancer rate that was 125 times higher than women who do not wear a bra! The kind of bra is not mentioned.

How long women wear a bra each day makes a major difference. "Women who wore bras for over 12 hours daily, have a 21-fold greater chance of developing breast cancer than do women who remove their bras before twelve hours." So there you have it ladies: when you come home from work, take off the bloomin' thing and celebrate your freedom! Why does that make me think of the movie *A Hundred and One Dalmations*, where at the end someone yells: *"Release the puppies!"*

And, now that we talk about bras: many modern bras are equipped with an iron or steel support around the cup. Could this be Victoria's secret? The steel wire not only functions as re-enforcement, but also as an antenna to all the different electromagnetic frequencies that we just talked about. The wire picks up the frequencies of radio, TV and telephone waves and transmits them to the delicate tissues inside the breast, which can become a cause of cancer as we have seen on the previous page.

Now don't y'all throw your bras away; just pull out the metal wire! And in case you wondered; no I've not yet heard of a twin set of breasts amplifying a local FM station! (Although I do know of a patient who could feel the telephone ring in her titanium total knee replacement.)

Did your doctor recently tell you again not to be in the sun for too long or not to go outside at all because of the risk of **skin cancer**? Well, science is saying the opposite!

A recent study found a significant correlation between cancer and a lack of sunlight. Five hundred and six regions in America were measured for ultra violet light. The regions with the lowest amounts of sunlight showed the highest amounts of cancer. The types of cancer that were found most were: breast, ovarian, and colon cancer.

So, too little light of the sun on your skin gives you a higher risk of contracting cancer.

It is said that too much exposure to sunlight on a sensitive skin can give you **skin cancer**. First of all notice that I wrote: too much!

Above the continent of Australia the ozone layer in space is the thinnest, which allows more radiation from the sun to reach us and we were not created to be exposed to this. Now does the sun cause skin cancer? It has not been proven as of yet. But I can imagine that the burning of skin by overexposure of sunlight together with the ingredients for cancer as we've discussed in chapter 2 can cause skin cancer. When all the cancer factors are present in your body and then you go out in the sun and get burned, the overexposure may trigger cancer of the skin, however it has not conclusively been proven!

What has been proven to be detrimental for your health is this: a lack of exposure to sunlight is related to deficiency in Vitamin D and that is related to higher rates of different kinds of cancer.

Vitamin D If you have cancer you need to know some more about vitamin D. And if you have black or dark skin you really need to sit up and take notes.

We're not going to talk about skin cancer anymore, from here on let's focus on the influence of sunlight and vitamin D on cancer in general.
- Less sunlight … less vitamin D … more disease.
- Less sunlight … more cancer.
- Less vitamin D … more cancer!

Most white people I know who have well-tanned skin are not sick or diseased. Most white people I know who are diseased have a very white skin and won't go out in the sun. I live in Florida, where many elderly people moved for the wonderful climate. Once they are here they try to stay away from the sun as much as possible.

Most African American folks who suffer from diabetes and other chronic diseases tell me they never go out into the sun. They have dark skin, which does not allow much light to penetrate through plus they hardly expose their skin to sunlight. A double whammy!

When a white person exposes eighty-five percent of his/her body to midday sunlight for twenty minutes, his/her skin will produce 1700 to 3400 International Units (IU's) of vitamin D.

After twenty to thirty minutes the skin stops making vitamin D, so longer exposure does not produce more vitamin D. Black people need to realize that their skin transmits less sunlight. They need three to six times more exposure to the sun than white skins (one to two hours.)

The RDA (recommended daily allowance) of vitamin D is set at 400 IU's by our government authorities. Researchers however claim that a higher dose is better, so many doctors nowadays recommend people to take at least 4000 IU's per day. Yes, that is ten times as much. You may think that that is too much, but wait. Tests have been done with daily amounts up to 500,000 IU's for three weeks showing no negative side effects. On the contrary; tests done with higher numbers of IU's all appeared to give more benefits.

Looking at these numbers I hope that you will realize that most of us will not get our fix of 4000

IU's per day, unless we spend time *daily* on the beach or near the pool in a bathing suit. Oh, and vitamin D can only be stored for sixty days in the body; so even a one week trip to Florida in the winter to load up on vitamin D does not cover you for the whole winter period.

Vitamin D, the sunshine vitamin, is making headlines these days:
based on a study of the data from 15,000 men over an 18 year study period, researchers from Boston's Brigham and Women's Hospital and Harvard Medical School concluded that men in this group who had the highest levels of vitamin D in their blood were 50% less likely to develop aggressive prostate tumors (the kind that kill.)

Most of us, especially people with darker skin are *deficient* in vitamin D and because of this we are more susceptible to disease in general and cancer in particular. The solution is simple. We'll have to help the sun a little and get additional vitamin D from other sources.

We can add organ meats, fish, eggs, butter, and raw milk to our diet and pop some extra fish oil capsules, but of course we can also supplement with Vitamin D tablets. They come in doses of 400 and even 1000 IU's.

When your pH is very low (4.5), be careful with **physical exercises**. Since you are suffering from a severe overload of acid, called acidosis, exercising your muscles will produce lactic acid, which will increase the acidosis and can make you feel bad. So, no heavy resistance exercises. Do not use weights.

Walking is a very healthy and natural way to use your muscles and cardiovascular system, as well as to get more oxygen in. When you walk, please do not use a "walkman," but try to get back in touch with nature, with your soul, your spirit and your creator. Take time to un-stress!

Many post menopausal women use some kind of **estrogen treatment** per doctor's prescription to avoid those nasty hot-flashes.

I found that many elderly women have been on estrogens for decades, but never skipped a couple of months to see if they still had the hot flashes.

As mentioned in Chapter 8, estrogens help to initiate the cancer process. When a woman is diagnosed with cancer, the first thing her doctor does is take her off all estrogens. Isn't that a suspicious practice?

Stay away from estrogens and progestins; they increase your chances of strokes, breast cancer and heart attacks! Try the pure and natural **progesterone** instead.

> "Progesterone has now been found to prevent and even control prostate cancer in men.-- (Dr. J. Mercola)

International authority on hormone treatment, Dr. John Lee, has a large number of anecdotal stories of complete reversals of metastatic prostate cancers. The clinical research on this has just begun. Dr. Lee stated that there are several studies that will be published in the near future confirming this observation in animal studies.

Hello, guys! Progesterone is NOT the hormone that makes guys grow boobs! It is the overabundance of estrogen_in our environment and diet that does this.

Ask your health-food store owner for the real progesterone and do not let any medical practitioner give you progestin, which is not the same as progesterone! (An excellent read for women is: *What Your Doctor May Not Tell You About Menopause*, by John R. Lee, M.D. and David Zava, Ph. D.; or ask for the Dr. Lee audio tape.)

> Looking for a more politically correct term for hot flashes?
>
> Just tell your husband next time you're sitting in front of the open fridge that you're:
>
> **"thermostatically challenged."**

An additional benefit of alkalizing your system is the following. According to Darrell Wolfe, a health practitioner, **obesity** is mainly caused by a system that is too acid. It is a scientific fact that *acid is stored in fat cells.* When the body is too acid, it tries to keep the dangerous acid away from the main organs, like the heart, the liver, etc. and it stores the acid in the legs. The more the acidity increases, the more fat cells are made and the heavier one gets. Consequently, alkalizing your body will take away the need for these fat cells and you may lose weight in the process!

Bee pollen helps the immune system. It is an excellent cell food and contains an excretion from the bees that help us fight tumors (from: *The Cancer Answer.*)

Add some **turmeric** to your food every day. It's a yellow spice that is known in India for its cancer preventative ability.

Old age is no excuse for disease. I hear many elderly folks say: "Oh, it's probably just old age!" Disease is not an inevitable part of growing old. According to the Bible we should live approximately a hundred and twenty years. It does not mention that the last part should be spent in misery.

A very likely cause for failing health at an older age is the sixty or seventy year long accumulation of toxins and depletion of minerals in the body. Often I hear people complain about their legs, and feet and toes in particular. They hurt, or they are numb, or the muscle strength is gone. There can be discoloration of the skin, or swelling with pain and the nails can get brittle. Some people have a whole variety of symptoms. The doctor cannot draw an accurate diagnose and there is no real treatment. What can you do?

Since the legs and particularly, the feet and toes, are furthest away from the heart, it does not take much imagination to figure that if there are toxins and sediment in the circulation, they will accumulate in those parts of the body where the blood flow is lowest and weakest – your lower legs and feet. Here the toxins and the slush will be found in highest concentration.

Can you still get these toxins out of your system? Yes you can! Even at an older age. By using a method called chelation.

The word **chelation** means *to grab*. Look for chelation treatment in your regular phone book and you'll find a clinic where you can go for treatment. You'll be examined by a medical doctor who will, through an IV (intravenous), connect you with a bag of chelating fluid that will drip into your bloodstream. The chelating substances "grab" the toxins and heavy metals and drop them off at your waste disposal organs: the kidneys and the liver. It takes about three hours per treatment, which you'll spend in a recliner, watching TV or reading a book.

It is a more than excellent way to get rid of toxins and heavy metals, especially when growing in age in a very toxic environment. The cost is approximately $ 90 per treatment.

You can even stay home and do the chelation yourself, by buying a product called "oral chelation" from Karl Loren or similar products. It is an excellent treatment!

> Chelation therapy has proven to reduce death rates from cancer by 90% compared to a similar group that did not get the chelation, according to Mr. Karl Loren, a scientist who worked as an adviser in the White House.

There are clear **dietary guidelines** in the Bible that were given to the people of Israel. They were written for their protection and well being. Science has confirmed again and again that these same guidelines will keep us from disease. They are:

- Do not eat blood or animal fat.
- Do not eat rabbit meat or pork. Even 'non Jewish' scientists have outlawed pork. It is full of toxins and parasites, which cannot be killed by cooking.
- Do not eat meat from predators; they accumulate toxins and pesticides in their tissues (alligator, shark, etc.).
- Any kind of fish that does not have scales or fins is "unclean." And for good reason! Catfish,

shark, eel, shrimp, shellfish and lobster all feed from the contaminated river and ocean floors and feed on cadavers. Ughhh! Think again when you order lobster, the ocean's giant cockroach.

Oh, and let's not blame God for our diseases. We all, in feeding our God given bodies, have "gone astray," and have served other gods. Our stomach, for one.

For years we have pounded our immune systems with junk food, toxins, heavy metals, etc. Unknowingly perhaps, but still. We've polluted our soil, our water and our air and live in a world of constant stress. For a while we get away with it and then suddenly we can fall ill and we blame God for it. We cry out "Why do You let this happen to me?" As if He loves to give us disease and make our lives miserable.

God is a good God. He was glad with the work of His hands. We messed it up. It is very healthy to take responsibility for your own health. As long as you blame someone else for your disease you can get stuck in apathy and bitterness, which have an acidifying effect on your tissues. Only when you own up to it, can you take new initiatives and choices to get back to wellness.

Once you are back to health again keep testing your pH every month. When you see your pH slide down, work your way back to where it is supposed to be; in the blue to dark green zone (6.5 – 7.0). It is easy to *maintain* the right pH. It is much harder to fight your way back out of the yellow or green; it can take months to get back into the right range.

Chapter 13

Did You Know That ...

The concept of **metastasis** or the spreading of cancer cells through the body by way of the blood and/or the lymph has never been proven to be true. It is just a theory. Hmmm ...! No cancer scientist has ever seen cancer cells in the arterial blood of a cancer patient. If that were true, every blood transfusion would have to be checked for active cancer cells. This, however, is not a standard procedure at the blood banks.

Medical science contradicts itself. Dr. R. G. Hamer has a different explanation for new cancers growing in other tissues of the body. The trauma of surgery or the mental shock of a dreaded diagnosis is the real cause of new cancer(s) springing up, according to Dr. Hamer. Animals, oblivious to a diagnosis, seldom show metastasis.

Dr. R. G. Hamer also holds that breast cancer is triggered by a separation or worry trauma in a woman's life, as in an abortion or a divorce. In case of an abortion or other loss of a child, a right-handed woman's left breast glands will be affected. The left breast is the primary nursing breast! (For a left-handed woman it is just the other way around.) Cancer of the right breast in a right-handed woman is caused by trauma through the loss of a *partner.*

More than fifteeen years ago the FDA found that ninety percent of the more than one hundred drugs they tested were still good beyond the **expiration date** and some for as long as fifteen years. So think again before you throw out your "old" stuff.

According to Gary Null Ph.D., and two other doctors, 783,936 Americans are killed each year by **modern medicine**. How many crashed 747's is that... per day?

Dr. Friedrich Douwes' **high temperature treatment** of a well-known German singer earned him a one-woman- musical dedicated to him and his staff, with tv crews and reporters present. After less than a year of high-body-temperature treatments for two hours every day, every sign of cancer was gone from her liver, ovaries, and lungs.

This hyperthermia treatment increases the circulation and probably supplies the tissues with an increase of oxygen. As you know by now, cancer and oxygen do not go together. So "sweat until they're dead.'"(cancer cells, that is).

In a study of 663 cancerous women who were treated with **needle biopsy** as a diagnostic tool, fifty percent were more likely to develop cancer of the lymph nodes in the armpit than those whose tumors were just removed.

If we may believe the media enormous numbers of people die each year of the flu. Want to know the real number? 240,000? 300,000? Less than a "whopping" one hundred seventy-five in 2005. Do you still feel that you need that flu vaccine?

Zyflamend, a new compound, added to a culture of human prostate cancer cells showed a seventy-eight percent reduction in the number of cells after seventy-two hours. It seems like the COX-2 inhibitors speed up the normal programmed cell death (apoptosis). Where do we find Zyflamend? In holy basil, turmeric, ginger, green tea, rosemary, oregano, scutellaria and hu zhang.

We all know that **lycopene** helps to fight cancer. *The Journal of Agricultural and Food Chemistry* found that organic ketchup contains one hundred eighty-three micrograms of Lycopene per gram of ketchup, compared to one hundred mcg's in non-organic brands. Fast food samples only had a poor sixty mcg's. The darkest red ketchup has the highest level of lycopene.

Instead of proving that sunlight causes skin cancer, scientists found that sunlight actually *prevents* **melanomas**. Vitamin D, the sunshine vitamin, contributed to a lower incidence of lymphoma (cancer of the blood). Men with the highest amount of vitamin D in their blood were fifty percent less likely to develop aggressive prostate tumors.

According to award-winning dermatologist Dr. Bernard Ackerman there is no proof that exposure to sunlight causes melanoma. One of his arguments is that the places where melanomas occur are hardly being exposed to sunlight: legs, torso, palms of hands and soles of feet.

Resveratrol, a substance in red wine is responsible for a fifty percent reduction in risk of prostate cancer. This stuff is also found in in peanuts and raspberries. Hallo: fifty percent! I hear ye! Nope, beer and liquors are *not* known for any significant benefits other than periodic happiness.

A study by the University of Hawaii concluded that a chemical added to **processed meats** like hotdogs, sausage, etc., is responsible for a sixty-seven hundred percent increased risk in pancreatic cancer. That is sixty-seven times. That is...very much!

If you have a family history of colon cancer you'll want to supplement with 400 micrograms of **folate** to cut your risk by fifty percent. Good sources for folate are spinach and asparagus.

Cancer cannot stand the (UV-) light of day! There is anecdotal evidence (by lack of expensive research program) that full spectrum light, or

daylight can stop and even heal cancer. Dr. Jane Wright, directing cancer research at Bellevue Memorial Medical Center in New York City in 1959, instructed cancer patients to stay outdoors as much as possible and to avoid being exposed to artificial light. The only patient who did not do better was...wearing glasses.

In an elementary school, in the Chicago area, all of the children but one were being taught in rooms where teachers kept the blinds drawn and the children were exposed all day to melanoma-promoting fluorescent light. The school reported five times the national average incidence of leukemia (cancer of the blood). When the teachers (what was wrong with them?) pulled the blinds up again the leukemia disappeared. We have light-sensitive glands behind our eyes that, apparently, need the good kind of (day-) light.

The frequencies of artificial lights are detrimental to our health. One wonders what the effect is of the light produced by computers, tv's and Play Stations. We may want to think twice about wearing (sun-) glasses too much. No facts were found yet on the use of contact lenses.

For those of you who live up in the northern regions where sunlight is hard to find, you'll be de-light-ed to know that there are full spectrum light bulbs for sale that can substitute for direct exposure to sunlight. It has also been found that sufferers of depression benefit greatly from a daily dose of full spectrum light.

Direct electric current has been used in medicine for many decades in orthopedic problems, in the treatment of pain and in regeneration of bone or other tissue to achieve faster healing. In Germany, direct current is used in cancer care by inserting needles near a tumor, but also by application on the skin. The object of using the current is necrosis (death) of the tumor cells, but ECT (electro cancer therapy) also induces a beneficial immune reaction and releases substances that help fight off tumor cells.

Now to all you "do-it-yourselfers": do not try out the current that comes out of the wall sockets in your house. Your home is hooked up to 110 volts, which is a killer and secondly, it is not direct, but alternating current.

Scientists in India discovered that **methylglyoxal** is so effective in targetting and killing cancer cells that eleven out of their nineteen patients who were in a very advanced stage of different kinds of cancer, returned to excellent health. This substance, when reaching the cancer cells, starves them to death very selectively. So normal cells are not affected. Sounds like a "silver bullet" to me! Hallo, Washington; are we researching this stuff already ...?

Ask your doctor why we're still doing chemo treatment and radiation.

A promising new technique is called **photo dynamic therapy (PDT)**. Light-activated drugs are distributed throughout the body and will concentrate in diseased tissue. A near-infrared laser light source illuminates the area which activates the drugs that kill the tumor tissue cells and stops the growth. A neat invention since it can "zap" the tumor that lives deeper in the tissues, like in the breast. No need for knife or needle! There are not many of these machines around yet, I'm sorry to say. Ask around!

Have you ever heard of **medical ghostwriters?** They're the Ph. D.'s who are hired by the pharmacomps to write drug reports that hype the benefits and hide the negative side effects, pocketing up to $20,000 per report. When completed, the drug companies then recruit real doctors to sign the reports with their names, which of course gives them instant prestige in the medical world when the reports are printed in peer journals.

Your family doctor cannot be blamed that he is taken for a ride. He is only following up on the latest information in his professional magazines, like every professional does. What's in it for you? You may end up with bad drugs disguised as good medicine. Beware!

In a recent newsletter from John Hopkins University we are warned about the chemical **dioxin**, a highly toxic and cancerous substance that is used in the fabrication of plastics. Do not use plastic containers or shrinkwrap in the microwave and do not store your waterbottles in the freezer.

The dioxin will be released in the water and drinking will be a hazard to your health! On the news you have probably seen shots of the Ukranian president Viktor Yushchenko who recently survived an assassination attempt with the same dioxin.

When you have been through surgery or you suffer from a heart condition, you probably had your doc put you on **coumadin or warfarin** for a while to keep your blood from clotting. Do you know that this stuff is also used as rat-poison? When rats eat too much of it they die of internal bleeding. When you're on coumadin your doctor will tell you that you cannot change your diet and especially not for the better! A sudden increase in your diet of healthy nutritious salads, for instance, would enrich your body with natural blood thinners which could make your blood too thin, with the risk of internal bleeding.

Aspirin is also used as a blood thinner and many of you have used a dose of eighty-one or three hundred twenty-five milligrams for years and years. Your doc assured you that it is completely safe and necessary. Well, he has to think again.

The University of Western Australia in Sidney studied one hundred eighty-seven patients who had been taking between seventy-five and three hundred twenty-five milli-grams of aspirin daily for more than a month. More than ten percent had developed little stomach ulcers, but only twenty percent of these folks experienced symptoms of the ulcers. After three months the researchers looked again in the stomach of the tested patients and found that seven percent had developed ulcers during this period. Aspirin safe ...? Think again!

Of course our question is: "Why not thin the blood with natural means that have no negative side effects?"

And often the answer you'll get is: there is nothing else! Well, yes, there is, but not in the form of a patented "drug."

There is fish oil and vitamin E, both having blood thinning properties. And there is natto, a natural product of steamed and fermented soy beans with a cheesy taste. It has been on the dinner table in Japan for many centuries. An enzyme derived from natto, called **Natto-kinase**, has been developed as a supplement that can be used successfully for circulatory problems. It has been used for over twenty years and is non-allergenic. Ask your health food store attendent.

Jill Siegfried, a University of Pittsburgh **lung cancer** researcher, holds that even if no American smoked, there still would be lung cancer, the fourth most commonly diag-nosed cancer. Makes you think if Dr. Hamer (Chapter 10) was right after all when he said that cancer is not caused by smoke but by a sudden psychological trauma. In the case of lung cancer it would be a sudden fear of death. Could it be the ultra violent movies that we are watching?

Do our bodies understand the difference between real death threats and the ones that Hollywood provide us with on a continuous basis?

Benzaldehyde is a chemical substance found in nature in many foods. It helps give coffee and cocoa their pleasant aromas, and is also widely used in the chemical industry. In the seventies Japanese scientists experimented with it and found it to be very effective in the treatment of cancer even in a very small concentration. Benzaldehyde is also one of the substances that make laetrile (Chapter 8) such a powerful cancer prevention agent. Why was it never published by the National Cancer Institute? Why is there no follow up research?

I told you to stay away from soda pop, right? The FDA states that **benzene** levels in bottled sodas increase after exposure to heat, light or just over time. In Britain more than twenty-five varieties of soda were pulled off the store shelves. Some contained more than thirty times as much benzene as is allowed in drinking water. The FDA did its own research here in the States. We're still waiting for the results…

In Washington there are twelve hundred registered pharmaceutical **lobbyists**. That outnumbers even the number of congress members they seek to influence. Hmmm…

Cherry farmers who up till recently advertised on the internet and informed people of the proven health benefits of cherries were warned by the FDA to stop it. In October, 2005, they received intimidating letters from the FDA. When cherry farmers disseminate their information, the cherries are being regarded as drugs, they wrote and of course we cannot have any of that...!

So the logic of the FDA runs kind of like this: when you say that something cures a disease it makes that something become a drug. Well then, if that something is a drug and you say that it cures a disease you must be a medical doctor, and if you're not a doctor you are practising medicine without a license, for which you can be locked up in jail.

If I claim that water can cure the medical condition called dehydration it makes water into a drug. And if I hand a bottle of water to a dehydrated person and say: "Here buddy, drink this and you'll get better!" I am practicing medicine without a license. I could end up in jail!

Beam me up, Scotty!

Lastly, just to show you that trying to find a cancer cure isn't always the work of top notch scientists and does not have to cost five million dollars up front; here is **Melanie Kabinoff** of fourteen years old, from Boynton Beach, Florida. Melanie became interested in curing melanoma to help her teacher who contracted the skin disease.

As a science project she exposed earthworms to UV-B radiation and then immersed them in five liquids with substances suspected of cancer curing properties: tea tree oil, vitamin D, coffee, soy milk and echinacea. After studying the effects of the fluids under a microscope, she found that tea tree oil and echinacea performed best. You rock, girl ..!

So this guy asks,
"Can I still get into heaven if I don't take minerals?"
And the answer,
of course is:

"Yes, and a lot quicker, too."

Chapter 14

The Future

The future isn't what it used to be. For decennia we looked to the future as the place and time where everything was going to be better, safer and healthier. Now that we live in it, where is it?

Where have all the promises gone about better and safer healthcare, less drugs, the victory in the war on AIDS and cancer, a more natural approach, better help from health professionals, and, most of all: more lives being saved through overall better health?

Although many surgical procedures and treatment technologies have improved over the years, people have not become happier with healthcare in general and with their doctor in particular. Ever since we have been promised that the "war on cancer" would be won in our lifetime, more people get cancer than ever before and more people are dying from it.

Where did we go wrong to believe that health is in a pill, an injection or a powder? A mistake was made at the onset of healthcare as we know it now – a mistake so big, it can be compared to building a skyscraper on the wrong foundation.

We'll need to go back in time to the second half of the nineteenth century, to find two French scientists: Louis Pasteur (we know him from Pasteur-ized milk) and Antoine Bechamp, both trying their best to influence the medical community of their time.

Pasteur had discovered that wine fermented due to the presence of bacteria. He discovered that heating the wine for a short while killed the bacteria in the wine, but did not deteriorate the quality of the wine. His theory was that germs are the cause of disease and that they can only manifest in one shape or form.

Bechamp, to the contrary, found that it was not the germ, or bacterium, that caused the disease, but that the state of the environment of the cell, or the inner body milieu, was responsible for changing a harmless germ into a disease-causing agent. He also found that ultra small micro-organisms can go through different stages of development and can evolve into various growth forms within their life cycles.

While Pasteur thought disease was caused by the aggres-siveness of the germ, Bechamp found that it was the lack of quality of the milieu that caused disease to happen.

Well, in school we all have learned about Pasteur. *His* name and *his* ideas became synonymous with health and disease. Bechamp however, ended up with the short end of the stick. Little do most of us know that Pasteur, on his deathbed, recanted his theory and admitted in one of his last breaths, that it was Bechamp who had been right all along.

Bechamp's idea that germs do not cause disease, but that they are the result of a *diseased milieu,* may at first look awkward but his conclusions were based on verifiable studies. He had found tiny particles in human blood that he called "microzyma." In our time and age they are called *micoplasmas.* Decades later these "micoplasmas" were made visible under special dark-field microscopes developed by a genius by the name of Royal Raymond Rife. The micoplasmas could be seen floating in the watery serum of the blood just like one can see the dust floating in the air when the sun shines its rays through a crack in the curtains of a dark room.

Rife observed that as the milieu, or environment changed, the micoplasmas changed, shifting from one form or shape into another and another. An astounding new discovery! What caused them to change?

When our blood or the fluid inside our cells has a pH of 7.4 they are in perfect balance and the micoplasmas live in harmony in and with the surrounding tissues. They are harmless. However when the pH drops they cannot thrive in the more acid environment and to survive, they will transform into another shape: a fungus, a virus, or ultimately into a bacteria. It is then that they can turn against us and make us sick. As a matter of fact; when the pH keeps dropping to the point where eventually death sets in, these bacteria, viruses and fungi will completely overwhelm us and consume and decompose the body, except for the bones.

The microscopic studies of R.R. Rife and G. Naessens have concluded that cancer is always found together with two micoplasmas. They have been called *markers* for cancer. And now you'll see how important the balance of the cell milieu really is and how essential it is to keep the pH exactly right.

> The slightest inconsistency in our tissue's pH can turn our tiny, harmless micoplasmas into disease-causing agents, attacking us from the inside out and overwhelming our immune systems.

So we can conclude that sickness is not per definition caused by ugly little monsters attacking us from the outside, but that the quality of the fluids and tissues inside our body is just as and perhaps even more important in keeping us healthy!

People with a proper overall body pH of around 7.1 just don't get sick as often and as severely as people whose pH has nosedived to lower values. Again, what went wrong?

The medical world chose Pasteur's model of disease and ridiculed any other idea (like homeopathy and chiropraxis). The enemy of health was an invader from outside the body that needed to be dealt with in the proper way. Research focused on finding ways to kill the invader through chemical means. Drugs were discovered to treat symptoms.

Treatment became very profitable. Drug producers formed cartels to protect and monopolize their business. Doctors were trained specifically and exclusively in the distribution of drugs. Politicians were lobbied. Laws were made and are being made that slam the doors shut to any other way of healthcare and to …cures.

Our medical professionals still do not look for answers in the right places. The directors of the American Medical Association can be blamed for ignoring cancer cures that scream at them in their faces. If they had listened and facilitated further research, cancer could have been eradicated by the 1940's. This atrocity is still being perpetrated on the American people until this very day. For instance, laetrile is still not for sale in the U.S.A. Another horrible example of how a ninety-nine percent successful *anti cancer vaccine* ends up in the dumpster can be read in appendix C. Read it and weep over America, folks!

Volumes can be filled with all the different discoveries that have proven successful in the real fight against cancer. These discoverers, these pioneers, are still being ignored by the medical establishment, and worse, by your government. Where are the people in government when they can do so much good for the people? They turn the other way while another ski trip or vacation ticket slides into their pocket. We're still on the wrong track of medication and profit.

There are other tracks where research has found, and still is discovering, very important and promising health solutions. Since so little is done to inform the general public about new approaches to healthcare, we'll spend some paper-space here to fill you in about one or two very important and very welcome new trends in healthcare. It will get pretty weird and I hope you will not throw this book into a corner now. Please hang on; it'll all make sense in the end.

14.1 Good Vibrations

When you have lived for more than 40 years on this breathtakingly beautiful blue planet called earth, you'll recognize the above heading as a song from the Beach Boys, but you most probably have not learned about the "quantum" theory in high school or college. Like me, you learned that the smallest possible particles in our universe are the electrons, the protons and the neutrons – the building blocks of the atoms.

Let's take a moment to put this in perspective and zoom in. The smallest particle of water that we can still call water is the water molecule.

A water molecule consists of two different atoms: a hydrogen and an oxygen atom. Going even smaller, these atoms consist of a center and one or more incredibly tiny particles that circle around the center. Inside the center we find the neutrons and the protons, but the electrons circle their way around with a speed that staggers the mind.

If, for a moment, we could shrink ourselves to atomic size and step inside one of the hydrogen atoms, we would be greatly surprised. Instead of seeing the substance hydrogen, we would see almost ...nothing. Hydrogen has a core consisting of two particles: a neutron and a proton. One electron is circling around the core. So here we are; inside the atom, standing next to the core, looking around us. The core of the atom is the size of two ping pong balls and the electron, the size of another ping pong ball, would be flying in a circle over our head on a distance of approximately one hundred fifty feet and with such a speed that we would not be able to see it! Two balls in the core and one ball at one hundred fifty feet distance with nothing in between. No air, nothing! So 99.9% of all the space that would surround us consists of ...nothing! Put that in your chewing tobacco and chew on it for a while!

Now let's un-shrink and get back to real size again; all the matter that we are so used to live with, the table, the wall, our car, our bones, it all is mostly ...nothing. The empty inter particle space takes up more than ninety-nine percent of all matter, so the book you're holding consists of ninety-nine percent of nothingness – just tiny vibrating bits that move so fast that we would not be able to even see them.

I promised it would get weird!

Albert Einstein, yep, the guy with the wild hairdo, had proven that the stuff we call matter is not really matter as we had imagined it to be, but that matter really is *a very condensed form of energy*. In other words, your chair, although it has the *appearance* of being solid matter on the macro (large scale) level, on the micro level only consists of compacted *energy*.

Some will say that your chair therefore is an illusion and that it's not real. Well, do not let your heart be troubled, I will stay on your side and say that your chair is a real chair and that everyone who believes differently is a cook.

What we get out of all this is a new understanding of creation and our physical universe. Things aren't just what they look like on the outside anymore. With this new knowledge we will have to widen our view of reality and perhaps we will grow in better understanding the world around us and inside of us. It will even broaden our understanding of the creator.

God is light. Light is energy. He created us in His image, which makes us energy beings. This helps me to get a more complete idea about spirit life and eternity and confirms the often heard statement that in this life we are spiritual beings undergoing a physical experience.

> When matter is condensed energy
> ...*we* are condensed energy.

That idea may be a shocker to you, but this new (quantum-) way of looking at things may be to our benefit. Like it or not, we live in an age where health researchers have begun to explore the wonderful world of "energy medicine" – the scientific study of how we can influence the vibrating microstructures of our bodies by other vibrations.

Without realizing it, you may have been treated already with an application of "energy medicine." Have you been to a physical therapist and treated with ultrasound for a painful tendonitis? The ultrasound head delivered energy with a particular frequency to your tendon tissue. The frequency was such that it increased the temperature in the tissue, which improved the circulation and shortened the healing time.

This treatment makes use of energy medicine. And think of all the diagnostic equipment that is based on the knowledge of energy medicine: x-rays, magnetic resonance imaging (MRI), cat-scan, ultrasound imaging, laser, etc.

Many folks have been successfully treated by an acupuncturist, who will look for spots of low resistance in your skin to add or rearrange energy to your body.

Perhaps you have had a moment of intense closeness with God, where you experienced a transfer of energy from Him to you, and found healing of your body or your emotions. It is very common and many people will tell you that they have this experience on a regular basis.

We can call this type of (Godly) energy transfer: *healing*. I hope this does not offend anyone believing in God. It should not diminish our experience with God in any way if we try to understand *how* He works in us. He still is the all mighty, unfathomable and powerful God, trying to communicate with us and to find resonance with us through His Holy Spirit. Often our receptors are not finding resonance with Him because of our busy lives or because we simply haven't yet tuned into Him.

Resonance takes place when two or more energy beings vibrate with the same frequency. When a tuning fork with the C key is hit and made to vibrate, it will cause the C string on a piano or guitar to vibrate with the same frequency. When this resonance takes place there can be a very easy transfer of energy between the two beings or objects – energy "flowing" from one to the other and vice versa. Remember the example with Ella Fitzgerald shattering a crystal glass in Chapter 4? Only when her voice reached the exact frequency of the crystal could she break the glass. When there is no resonance, the energy transfer stops or is much slower.

If we may believe the scientists, the people who have explored our world on a micro level, we and the entire material world around us are energy beings, all vibrating with our own particular, personal frequencies. Our cells vibrate each with their own distinct frequencies. A group of cells, as in the liver, will vibrate with a different frequency than a bone or an earlobe, or a whole body. Each person, being a totality of trillions of cells, will vibrate with his or her own frequency signature. Any added frequency will change and influence the total sum.

A medication can calm us down or fight an infection. The new frequency of the medication or herb added to the frequency of a sick person can change the frequency of a certain diseased part of the patient's body.

Dr. Hulda Clark's "zapper" works in the same way. The added frequency range will somewhere in our body find a parasite and be in resonance with it. The transfer of the energy of the electric power to the parasite is too much for it and it will vibrate to …death. Goodbye, parasite!

In homeopathy the beneficial frequency of a specific herb is, by continued shakings of the bottle, passed on to the water in the bottle. This water, when taken as medication, delivers the frequency of the herb to the tissue in need of it.

With our voice too we can cause changes in our physical bodies by finding resonance with other people's voices, for instance when we sing together. This can make us feel good and calm us down. We have exchanged energies.

A wonderful book is *The Hidden Messages In Water*, by Masaru Emoto (Chapter 5). The author took pictures of frozen water molecules that formed beautiful crystals. When the water was exposed to blessings that were spoken in the presence of the water, the water crystals were of great beauty, but when curses were spoken the water often could not form even a poor crystal. It seems like water is influenced by the frequencies we send out with our voices. We are seventy percent water!

In prayer we also search for resonance with God's Holy Spirit to find calmness, rest and oneness. He takes our burden, which we can call *negative energy,* and fills us with wholesome energy, or power.

I hope that by now you have a more practical idea of what it means when we say that we are energy beings. We and everything around us are constantly being affected by a continual exchange of cascading, flowing and vibrating energies.

I know, for most of us all the above is simply too hard to fathom. Going through high school and college we had a vague idea of what matter was all about and we went on living our lives. Science had figured out just about every-thing that needed to be figured out. We got married, had a couple of kids and told our ten year-olds with blissful ignorance about the exciting world of atoms and electrons. We were happy, life was simple! Then came this quantum energy theory, messing up our whole idea about life and throwing us all off balance.

There is more...

There is another outburst in research that, if ignored, will limit your understanding of what is taking place in the more holistic range of healthcare. (Holistic means: the total man/woman, body, soul and spirit) We need to talk about *electromagnetism*!

I'm sure you have seen a magnet before with a north and a south pole and the magnetic lines making a visual pattern in a layer of iron dust. When you take away the iron dust the invisible magnetic field lines are still there all around the magnet. These field lines extend outwardly until infinity; they form an invisible pattern, or **field** all around the iron core.

Any machine that generates electricity also has field lines that circle around the wire coil because the electric current (a stream of free flowing electrons) in the wires induces the magnetism. It also has its own field.

On a micro level *all matter* produces magnetic field lines since all matter consists in part of circling, moving electrons.

The movement of electrons produces magnetism and magnetism in turn affects the flow or current of electrons. They both interact and influence each other continually! The field takes up a three dimensional space extending in and around the core.

You too have an invisible field. Isn't that cool? The mass of moving electrons in your body produces a magnetic field that is measurable up to a few feet beyond your skin. Fields interact with each other when they overlap, because their field lines influence each other electromagnetically.

Moving your field lines through another field changes the flow of electrons in that field; and the changed flow of electrons produces an altered, new field. Fields are continually changed by a whirlwind of these power lines crisscrossing their space. This could very well be what love and attraction is all about. When two people who are in love snuggle up to each other their fields overlap and intermingle, producing desirable feelings and happiness.

So, when our field is being changed ...we change! Let's go a little further with this: When I think a certain thought I cause nerve impulses to cascade back and forth between different parts of my brain and so I change the flow of electrons, or current, in my brain, right? This change of electrical current causes an electro-magnetic change in my field, right? That is *my* field, right?

When I think and produce thoughts, I am changing my own personal field which in turn influences the electron flow in my body which causes electrical, magnetic, and chemical changes and probably a whole lot of other things that we have never even thought about. When I think about my wife it can cause me to get butterflies in my stomach; it literally changes my chemistry, which in turn changes my mind and influences my actions. I'll go buy her flowers.

That is the message we need to remember: we have and we are a field. This field is influenced by invisible energy forms like electricity, magnetism, frequency waves from who knows what (radio, TV, cell phones, microwave equipment, your electric blanket, the sunlight, etc.). All these changes in my field will have an impact on my physical being: my body, my mind and my chemistry.

The Future

Hesitantly, without any certainty, I step out and dare to call this field: my ...*spirit*. Could it be that in our time and age, probably without even realizing it, we are discovering something more of what we have always called: the spiritual world?

Could it be that my field is that dimension of myself where creativity, ideas, believe, faith and love originate? Is this the realm where my intuition is sparked? Is it here where I can sometimes sense God's presence? Does His Holy Spirit find resonance with me in this invisible field-space of mine? Is my conscience impregnated here in this field with either good thoughts or bad ones? I leave you to answer these marvelous questions for yourself.

Where healing of cancer and other diseases is concerned, our fields may very well be the place where healing either is received, or where the motivation to want to be healed (prayer) is formed. And then, my friends, these new ideas and thoughts become a new ocean to sail on.

I hope I did not write anything here that might be offensive to you.

Many Christians who are being confronted with these new insights will label them "new age" and, being afraid for the unknown, will not have anything to do with them. I do not agree with them for the following reasons: These new insights are not a new theology; they are new ideas about how creation works and interacts. The tools of science have improved since we were in high school; you and I should expect new theories and ideas about reality from scientists.

Modern research has stepped over the boundaries that were limiting us a decade ago. They and we have stepped into a new realm, or dimension, where things are so small that we cannot see them anymore. We try to imagine what reality is like in this micro-cosmos, but often we just can't! However, these new discoveries of our God-given reality need to be integrated in a new worldview and also in a more complete understanding of who we are. We should not leave this to those who do not know God.

New Age fills up the space that is left empty by Christians who are afraid to tread into these new territories of science. If we, the followers and believers of Jeshua, hesitate to give meaning to the latest research and discoveries, we swing the doors wide open for the followers of paganism (New Agers) to write the headlines in our children's school books!

How can a scientist fathom the wonder of a water crystal perfected by an expression of love, if he does not know that God made Himself known to be a loving God? Creation per definition expresses God. So far I have not found anything in the discoveries of science that has limited my concept of who God is; it only has grown by leaps and bounds.

Being a Christian myself and trying to familiarize myself with the research in these new fields of study, I've come to realize more and more the vastness, the all-pervasiveness and omni-presence of our creator and God. The God of the Bible has even become closer to me; being more than ever aware of His spirit (His field) seeking resonance with little me and my spirit (my field) to teach me, bless me and to do His bidding here on earth. I hope you will be able to share this with me.

Chapter 15

A Phantom in the Cell Milieu

In Chapter 1 we saw that we can start to talk about cancer when a perfectly normal healing/repair process, where new cells are made, is not inhibited and stopped when the repair is completed. The "command" for the repair process is probably given by estrogens when toxins, trauma and radiation are damaging our tissue cells. Dr. Hamer showed us in Chapter 10 that our brain and our mind are involved in this command process as well. Apparently, even the fear of, or the threat of damage can initiate the repair process as if the brain anticipates it and the brain can also shut down the repair after the trauma (DHS) has been resolved and the threat is not experienced as such any longer.

The trouble starts when the necessary ingredients for the inhibition of the repair process are absent! We saw that *laetrile* has to be present at the repair site to stop the growth action. But since laetrile has disappeared out of our diet (and since the FDA has taken it out of our shops) we have become vulnerable and the normal repair processes that are going on in our body are not being stopped every time they happen. The "Super-Growth"-cells and the normal cells keep piling up and form a large group of cells: a tumor. Only now can we start speaking of having cancer!

Anything that switches on the repair process by some-how damaging our tissue cells can end up in a tumor? Well, yes, laetrile is the main doorkeeper, we could say, but there is more going on.

In the previous chapters we have seen enough evidence to say that tumors will only grow when the involved cells are in poor condition and that cancer can only survive in an acid, oxygen-deprived environment. So the cell's condition and its environment are important factors in the growth of cancerous tumors.

All these factors have to come and conspire *together!* Even if one factor is taken out of the equation it can mean a stop to cancer. For instance, I hope you remember that Dr. Budwig's recipe, in Chapter 6, by itself gave many people back their health and life.

There is one cancer-factor we have not talked about yet. Sorry, but I first had to bring you up to speed on mico-plasmas and energy medicine in the previous chapter.

In 1934 cancer patients were healed from their cancers in clinical studies at the University of Southern California. Royal Raymond Rife, a tenacious scientist, built a micros-cope that could enlarge to a degree that, in that time, was thought to be impossible. With this scope Rife could see *living* viruses inside cells. It had never been done before! The later built electron microscope could only see dead viruses.

Rife discovered tiny parts of viruses floating in the fluid of the cell that could shift shape like the Phantom of the Opera. One moment they could be seen while a moment later they simply disappeared out of sight.

As we've seen in Chapter 14, Rife had found the mico-plasma (which can be regarded as a tiny virus) and with this discovery he had proven that Antoine Bechamp's theory was right after all. One of these micoplasmas he called BX. It was found consistently in the presence of cancer. Rife discovered that BX could be killed by a specific frequency and so he developed an electric frequency generator that specifically targeted the BX micoplasma. (The machine was about 3 feet high, which is of Frankensteinian proportion if you compare this generator with Hulda Clark's small, handheld, Zapper.)

The machine worked wonderfully well. People were cured; yes, *cured!* Rife became famous; the medical doctors who partook in this undertaking wrote their theses and cancer was eradicated… Well, not so fast; yes, people were healed, but when that happened, representatives of the AMA stepped in and tried to buy Rife out. Rife refused because he knew what would happen. As always, when fortunes can be made, there are vultures circling the prey. Rife wanted his discovery to benefit mankind and he knew that his technology was not welcome in medicine land and would probably end up in the basement, never to be used. He was right.

When Rife refused he was sued for practicing medicine without a license – the old trick that works so well for the pharma-comp dominated AMA and FDA. Rife was sued and his office was ransacked and burned. His technology, his books and his research went up in smoke. Yes, you can blame the death of your loved ones who died from cancer to these fascist authorities of the AMA and the jerks in government who connived with them. *Are you getting mad yet …?*

What is left from Rife's discoveries is the following: His technology is being rediscovered by independent scientists, who of course are helped by the latest technologies. Electrical frequency generators are being made with more and more sophistication. I told you about the zapper, but there are different generators that can zoom in on very specific frequencies. The zapper can be purchased with a cancer-specific key that generates only cancer related frequencies.

Although I could not find proof of people having been directly contaminated or infected, Rife and others have found the cancer virus/micoplasma to be present in mushrooms, chicken and other meat but specifically in pork.

A Phantom in the Cell Milieu

One of Rife's contemporaries was Dr. Livingston-Wheeler, who developed a vaccine for the cancer virus and treated herself with it. She too was ridiculed by the powers that be of her time.

Gaston Naessens, with a self-built microscope, found the same virus as Rife. Naessens was thrown out of France and does further research in Canada.

Sam Chachoua recently developed a cancer vaccine and, again, lost all his material to the powers that be. His vaccine is available. Read his story in Appendix C!

In the previous chapter we learned that viruses, or micoplasmas, shift- shape dependent on the pH of the fluid they are in. In an alkaline solution micoplasmas tend to take on the smallest form or even disappear under the radar screen altogether. In this form they are not known to play a role in cancer. However when the fluid is more acid and has a lower pH, the micoplasma will take on a larger form, which is recognized as the BX cancer-marker in cancer tissue.

It is not known what kind of role the BX micoplasma plays in the cancer cell. Rife said: "In reality, it is not the micoplasma that produces the disease, but the chemical constituents of these micro-organisms enacting upon the unbalanced cell metabolism of the human body that in actuality produce disease. We also believe, if the metabolism of the human body is perfectly balanced or poised, it is susceptible to no disease."

So, yes, we can do something! We can prevent the mico-plasma from shifting to a larger, cancer-marking form by keeping our body in balance, or, if we have cancer, we can force them back into hiding by re-alkalizing our cells.

The *collagen* of connective tissue can be made to shift shape just like the micoplasmas by heat! Possibly, by turning up the body heat by inducing fever, we may also see the micoplasmas shift back into hiding. Perhaps this is the dynamic of hyperthermia treatment mentioned in Chapter 13.

And lastly, as we've discussed before, viruses do not like oxygen. Well-oxygenated tissue may be your best defense against micoplasma activity.

Dr. Livingston-Wheeler treated more than 10,000 cancer patients from 1968 to 1983 in her clinic in San Diego, showing a 80% success rate. Anyone reading this must think: *she must have been doing something right!* In 1971 Richard Nixon signed a $ 1.6 billion "war on cancer" into law. Of course you would like to know how many millions of dollars were used for new research to follow up on her success. The answer? Zilch, nada, nothing!

Not a penny.

Now, I trust, you're really mad.

Chapter 16
Treating, Curing, Healing

Now that we're wrapping up the stream of information in this book, what is the big picture that we can carry with us into the future?

We've looked at the cancer factors, the milieu, the triggers, oxygen, water, the immune system, the parasites, acidity and the micoplasmas. You've read a stack of information that was verified by doctors and scientists. You know a lot more and I hope that by now you feel empowered. Although cancer has reached epidemic proportions in our lifetime, cancer can be beat!

Our culture is conspiring against the consistency of our cell's milieu and our health in general. Every effort is thrown at us to entice us to lower the pH of our milieu and become vulnerable to disease: coke, coffee, alcohol, white bread, tons of meat, some more coke, mayonnaise, cigarette smoke, no exercise, stress, a doughnut, chewing gum, another coke, margarine, and lots of empty water. When we finally drag ourselves to the doctor he gives us, to top it off, one or two new medications, that are very acidifying as well – and perhaps a diagnosis that blows a fuse in our mind and triggers fear, anxiety and more stress.

While increasing in age, many people find themselves on the slippery slope of their body's pH scale, slowly sliding to the acid side and falling into the hands of the pharmacomps.

Disease sets in and the doctor prescribes a medication, which, in nearly all cases, helps you to cope with the *symptoms* of the disease such as pain, depression, sleeplessness, tumors, anxiety, hot flashes, higher blood pressure, a raised cholesterol level, etc. Although you may feel better for a while the side effects of the medication will eventually manifest in *new symptoms*. Anti-cholesterol meds can give the side effects of muscle wasting and worse: death. Pain meds often give such constipation that people need stool softeners, another, *new medication!*

You get more and more symptoms, which results in more and more med's, which come with more and more side effects that need more and more meds and doctor visits. It all looks like a juggler's stage act where you are the juggler assisted by doctors trying to keep more and more saucers (symptoms) spinning on their sticks, running from one to another to keep the show going, while your assistants add more saucers behind your back. This is called...treatment!

The symptoms are the outward appearance of what is really happening inside your body on a *cellular* level. If only we could fix the problem on the cellular level we could skip the whole juggler's act. Then the disease would be cured!

I can remember our family doctor (just one!) coming to my parent's house to visit me as a child because I had bronchitis. He would come and sit with my mother and me to find out what I was eating and drinking, take my vital signs and take the time to "get the whole picture." He would be there at least twenty minutes to drink coffee and advise my mother to keep track of my temperature. He did not want to give me antibiotic medications because he said it was better for me to build up resistance to the disease. My doctor was dedicated to *curing* me instead of *treating* me.

He passed away many years ago. Those days are over, folks! We're talking managed care now, boy! How much time do you spend with your doctor? Five minutes? Ten? Fifteen? I recently visited a lady who was on twenty-seven medications. She asked me why she had all these symptoms; pain, muscle spasms, nausea, headaches, etc. The stack of papers that explained all the side effects of her meds was as high as this book is thick.

How can we expect a doctor to oversee and monitor all these meds, all these side effects and the multiplied bad interactions of all these drugs with each other, while having to be ready for the next patient in fifteen minutes! He simply cannot!

Treatment:
- focuses on symptoms not the cause,
- often adds more symptoms,
- strongly acidifies the body,
- is very, very expensive,

- does not cure the disease,
- is very time consuming.

As we've seen in previous chapters the medical system is geared for treatment since continuous treatment generates continuous profit. From a business standpoint we have to conclude that the healthcare system in America, next to the oil companies, is probably the best profit generating system ever.

Supply and demand are completely and rigorously controlled and manipulated, from the patient who needs a band aid to the president who needs pharma-money to buy himself into the White House after which he signs bills that further strengthen the drug business.

The diseased people merely exist as conduits in this system and are disposable. I realize that sounds crass, but I dare you to read Appendix C: "A horrible, horrible story."

I do not want to judge the people who are in authority over this system; they will have to answer for their responsibilities to a higher power. But we have to conclude that our health system is rotten to the core and that it is the biggest obstacle in the search for bona fide cures for cancer and other diseases.

More and more people are realizing that if they hand over the responsibility for their health to a doctor they will receive treatment, but if they want to be cured they need to start taking responsibility for their own health. This is an excellent trend! A cure is aimed at fixing the problem; it has no side effects, raises the body pH back to normal values, focuses on nature and often is much cheaper than treatment.

Every doctor worth his salt will tell you that the only one able to cure is the body itself. If we give the body what it needs it will heal itself. Unless there is genetic damage every body is designed and equipped to seek and facilitate its own repair. It is our responsibility to make sure the body has all the necessary ingredients (nutrients) to make and keep health possible.

It means eating the right foods and drinks in the right amounts and staying away from contamination by toxins like heavy metals and refined oil products and making the body function in a natural way; for instance walking.

Even when doing the best we can, we still breathe in heavy metals from engine combustion and garbage disposal plants. We use chemicals in our shampoo, toothpaste, dental work, laundry detergent, etc.

We need to become more aware of our environment and we simply have to do the best we can! While we're doing that, we should try to stay away from doctors and hospitals. Not because doctors are evil people, but they are the well meaning representatives and facilitators of an evil system and the risk factor of you being killed by a wrongly prescribed medication or a contaminated hospital ward is very high.

Patients in this country received the wrong medication, inaccurate or delayed test results, and improper treatment thirty-four percent of the time.

> According to Gary Null, Ph.D., and others: "The number of *unnecessary* medical and surgical procedures performed annually is 7.5 million. The number of people exposed to *unnecessary* hospitalization annually is 8.9 million. The total number of deaths inadvertently induced by a physician or surgeon or by medical treatment or diagnostic procedures is *783,936.*"

In addition it needs to be mentioned that most medical errors go unreported, which may even double the number.

Again, that is more than 783,000 deaths by medical mistakes, which makes the American medical system the leading cause of death and injury in the U.S.A. Our medical system should be first on the danger list of Homeland Security!

The FDA, the officials who were installed to protect the American public from those vested interests are heavily involved as well. Nobody is looking out for you and me anymore. It is a scary situation, where money hungry corporations and politicians are preying on an unsuspecting population driven from one scare to the next health hoax and paying dearly for it with tax dollars.

Do you realize the tricks they are playing on you? Do you understand that when your president allocates $100 million for AIDS relief in Africa he basically writes a check to Bayer or MS&D for $100 million to dump their overstocked and often outdated AIDS medication on the African continent? Yep, that's *your* tax money.

And how much have they, in cooperation with the media, scared you into believing that the next anthrax or Avian-flu is going to kill you and your family if you do not get vaccinated in time? So our government buys hundreds of millions of dollars worth of vaccines to stockpile for possible epidemics that may never come about.

Remember the anthrax scare? Well did it ever come to an epidemic? How many people died? Three? And how much money on tax dollars went to the pharmacomps?

The educational systems, your government officials, the news media, the defense department, most of the cancer research, and the pharma-comps are in it for money, prestige and power. They do not seek to cure you of your disease. Your disease is their target for financial success and they are very determined to keep things exactly the way they are.

In January '05 thirteen-year-old Katie Wernecke, when diagnosed with cancer of the lymph nodes, was taken from her parent's home by the state of Texas against the family's will, who tried to protect her from the radiation treatment that the medical powers had ordained. Her mother was arrested and her three brothers were placed in a foster home. The parents were labeled neglectful. They only wanted her daughter to be treated with intravenous vitamin C, by a physician, which has been documented as a very successful treatment for many diseases.

This case shows you how medical professionals are able to enlist the help of government agencies in order to *force* people into medical treatments that can actually pose significant health dangers. Our government is not on our side anymore. Our freedom has been lost!

Internationally the pharmaceutical industrial powers are well on their way towards legislation that will cover not only all medications under prescription, but also all supplements and herbs (the "Codex Alimentaris"). It means that if these powers are not being driven back, soon you will pay double for your vitamin C after you've also paid your co-pay for an extra doctor's visit to get the prescription.

Their aim is total world control over healthcare, food industry and distribution of goods and services.

And here comes the really scary part: these ultra-rich industrials (let's call them a cabal), who have their tentacles in every layer of government also have very straightforward ideas about world population control.

For years our Pentagon, has done research on how disease can be used as a weapon. The motive? The Russians did it and "we could not stay behind."

Remember the micoplasmas? Because of their size they are not detected in normal blood and tissue tests as causes for disease. They would make excellent stealth weapons of mass destruction, transported in warheads or used in airplane aerosols, carried around in a lady's purse.

Many reports have been written about the Pentagon doing tests with pathogenic (disease-causing) micoplasmas with population groups and whole cities in the U.S.A. and Canada, (Winnipeg, Manitoba in 1953; Punta Gorda, Florida in 1957).

OK, you'll say; what does all this has to do with me fighting my way back to health? Well, as long as you have the expectation that our medical system will take care of you and your family, this system will continue and your children and grandchildren will die from diseases that should have been eradicated years ago. As long as we expect to be cured by this cabal, we will stay in the same rut and nothing will change for the better. We will stay diseased, we will continue to spend kazillions of dollars, insurance will go up and up, and we will get more and more frustrated, seeing our loved ones die under the care of our medical system.

First of all we should expect our representatives in government to come with legislation that will make an end to the stronghold of the pharma-comps and that will redirect money towards development of cures. This by itself probably will take nothing less than a revolution.

We should expect scientists to come up with cures, which will only happen if our government will give them a budget and then will leave them alone and let them do their jobs. Scientists love to find cures, if we let them. The space program is a fine example.

Doctors, many of whom started off as humanitarians, would love to be involved in curing patients, if only the American Medical Association and the FDA would back off and let them. We need statesmen, not politicians, of whom we can expect to right the wrongdoings of the governmental agencies that have run amuck. We should expect to eradicate cancer, MS, lupus, diabetes and a host of other diseases in perhaps less than ten years. Most of the groundwork has been done already.

The billions of dollars wasted on unnecessary and dangerous drugs could be reallocated towards health insu-rance for everyone. We should also expect government to close the gate to frivolous law suits. Lawyers should be redirected to their right place in society instead of preying on mishap and mayhem, cranking up the cost of just about everything in life. Our nation could once more become a blessing to a world in suffering and …still safe money.

Until that day arrives we are in danger and we need to cover our backs and our health. Beware of when, how and how much to expose yourself to all the technology that this perverted healthcare system has to offer you.

We don't think much of having an x-ray taken of our chest or breast. Media are telling us we need to be screened for TBC and for breast cancer. What we do not hear is that x-ray exposure is by itself a cancer trigger. Oh, and your yearly flu shot? Have you checked with your doctor lately what is *in* that vaccine? No? Well, nine out of ten he does not know either! Do you realize that the only thing your doctor knows about the drug he or she prescribes to you is what the pharma sales rep is parroting to him/her? That sales rep has no degree in biology or medication – only a training in sales techniques!

So how *do* you know if that vaccine is safe? What about the heavy metal stabilizers like mercury that have to be added to the vaccine cocktail to keep it from going stale? The answer is you don't know and neither does your doctor!

Vaccine exposure has become a very dangerous, unaccep-table risk and has been indicated as a way of infection transfer, causing even new diseases like Autism, AIDS, creutzfeldt-jakob syndrome and fibro-myalgia, of which most of these are believed to even have been developed and created in laboratories hired by the Pentagon. Hallo! That's your tax money at work! You have to look out for yourself like never before.

Do not fall for just any treatment that is offered to you when you find yourself diseased. Remember that thousands of people have been killed by taking vioxx, prozac or hormone replacement therapy – drugs that were approved by the FDA!

Find a physician who does his homework in keeping up to date with the latest research. Find one with an open mind to alternative, natural treatment and a healthy reserve against medications. Make sure he or she takes enough time to listen to you when you share your health history. Ask for his credentials and look up his name on the Internet. It is important to know who your doctor really is. He or she will be the person you are going to trust your health and wellbeing to!

Your doctor may not have the same cultural background. In my work I meet doctors from India, Pakistan, China, the Philippines and the Middle East. I'm sure they are very capable and talented and I will trust them fixing my broken leg or implanting an artificial joint.

For the physical aspects of my health and in seeking treatment and even a cure, I can work together with a Chinese herbalist or a Taoist acupuncturist. Although they are from a different culture and belief system I can benefit from their skills and know how.

It becomes a totally different matter when I seek my *healing*.

While treatment and cures take place at the physical and mental level, for *healing* we need to open up another dimension, the spiritual dimension. Healing includes every aspect of us. Body, mind *and spirit*.

In this new stressful millennium our spirit, that was meant to be in perfect relationship and resonance with the Creator of the Universe, is often underdeveloped, atrophied and filled with garbage. And with the depletion of our spirit our sense of direction, our intuition, our worship has ceased. We have lost spiritual properties that we desperately need back to stay healthy or to regain our health. More and more we can read about scientific research that confirms the connection between prayer and health. But besides the science of it, we all know very well that our spirit needs to be in synch with the rest of us and with our Creator.

Healing requires not 'just' the repaired cooperation in and between the cells of body parts, like liver, lungs, muscles and brain. It necessitates resonance between the whole person and his or her Maker on a spiritual level. And finding this resonance demands a choice that every one has to make sooner or later.

I have made that choice years ago and that is why I strongly recommend your doctor to be a person who has a personal relationship with the God of the Bible. Only a doctor who can relate to me as a fellow Christian can assist me spiritually in my personal quest for wholeness.

Read the books! An acid *body* is often caused by a *mind* that worries, hates or is not loved. When disease sets in it can be reversed by treatment or a cure, but the *reoccurrence* of disease can only be completely erased when the whole man or woman has been made well; and that means when the *spirit* has been brought to life and has been healed.

A healed spirit is the most powerful source of strength and wholesomeness, folks, because it enables us to reconnect with the ultimate healer, the Creator. He has made a way to connect with Him again. His spirit seeks to connect with our spirit to have *resonance*. That can only happen through a conduit, whose name is Jeshua. Read more about it in the new testament of a book that is still on the bestseller list: the bible.

Harmony in body, soul and spirit will keep us in good health!

Read, read, read and spend much time in health food stores. Become informed in the different products. Read labels like you never did before!

Be extremely delicate in keeping your cell milieu clean and alkaline. Stay away from processed foods, toxins, heavy metals and petroleum products if you can. Do not allow stress, hate or depression. Do not allow your pH to sink to acid values. Guard your spirit. Take responsibility. Look out for yourself. Take some vitamin C every hour. Pray! Feed your body! Rest your soul and spirit! Take off on Sunday or another day. Really off! Fill your *Field* with healthy, wholesome reality, not with the *second hand experiences* of the actors of the silver screen. Speak health to your body! Bless it! Live in moderation. Walk every morning and evening. Ask Christians to soak you in prayer daily. Express love. Hug a cashier. Enjoy the present; it still is the first day of the rest of your life. Read this book again. Give some of your money to the poor every week and enjoy the giving. Practice laughing out loud in the car. Take your minerals! Be happy with what you see in the mirror even if it wears a hair piece or a temporary wig. Make restitution to anyone you owe money or love. Be proud of your skin even if it sags; it is *your* skin. Love everybody! Even Hitler had a mom. Try every week if you can still stand naked upside down on your bed. Laugh hard and often, mostly about yourself. Live righteously but do not take yourself too seriously; nor your disease. Give your tumor a name and tell 'Fred' that although you love him it is better for both of you that he leaves right now. Plant a sun flower. Be a volunteer Wal-Mart greeter. Join a church choir. Feed the birds. Listen to beautiful music. Be honest. Direct an orchestra in your bathroom with real loud music. Read a psalm. Tap away your hang ups and pain with EFT. Make peace with everyone. Soak your feet in Epsom salts together with a neighbor. Be nice to all. Talk to God. Sing loudly in the shower, then talk some more with God. Tap some more and take some more minerals. Never curse. Love and obey God and, finally, make sure you're on the right side of eternity when you end up on the wrong side of the grass. The certainty of a future with God makes the present bearable and even enjoyable.

God bless' you!

Appendix A

Emotional Freedom Technique

*"The cause of all negative emotions
is a disruption in the body's energy system."*
-- Gary Craig

We have all grown up with a rough notion about what psychology and psychiatry are all about. We may not understand all the cleverly designed ideas from "shrinks" like the proverbial doctor Sigmund Freud, whose "invention" of the psychiatrist's couch we remember from movies of Alfred Hitchcock and others. Still we all seem to understand that deep down under the surface of the human conscience lingers a vast and unknown waste land of forgotten memories: the unconscious.

It is the job of the psychiatrist to help us dig up stuff from the unconscious that causes us to stagnate in our present functioning. Negative emotions have their roots in things that happened in the past and that have become unconscious to us. The trick is to make them conscious again, relive the experience and find a better response to it. That is the general idea.

Is it the right idea? Does it hold water? Has it proven itself? Well, it has helped some, but the overall poor results of psychiatry speak for themselves.

In our endeavor to overcome cancer, we do not have the luxury of a two-year-long series of therapeutic sessions to uncover the cause of anxiety or worry. We need a solution now and it has to stick! So let's turn away from the conventional way of dealing with feelings and thoughts and let's look at it from an entirely different angle.

According to modern science, man can be understood as an energy being. All the atoms of our body are in constant vibration, taking up and giving off energy every split second of our life. These different energies connect through certain pathways. An example of this is the massage therapist who applies pressure to certain points of the foot to ease a headache, or an acupuncturist who puts energy in the form of a hot needle in part of the ear to treat a condition of the kidneys.

To most observers who have grown up and were educated in Western culture, this practice does not make sense at all. What has the foot to do with the head, or what has the ear to do with the kidney? To the massage therapist and the acupuncturist however it does make sense, because he or she has seen the good results. These results have brought these energy medicine practices into the public spotlight in the last decade.

Although we do not know exactly how all these energy therapies work or how these systems are connected, the results are there to show that they work. (More about energy medicine in Chapter "The Future.")

We can be sure of one thing: the future of medicine is for those scientists who pursue the knowledge and understanding of these new energy medicine principles.

It was Dr. Roger Callahan, who, by coincidence, found out that "tapping" on certain places of the body, while focusing on an emotional problem, gave almost immediate relief of anxiety symptoms.

Here is how he found out. In 1980, Dr. Callahan was working with a patient, Mary, for an intense water phobia (fear). She suffered from frequent headaches and terrifying nightmares, both of which were related to her fear of water. To seek help she had been going from therapist to therapist for years, with no substantial improvement. Callahan tried to help her with conventional means for a year and a half. He did not make much headway either. Then one day he stepped outside the normal boundaries of psychotherapy. Out of curiosity he had been studying about the body's energy system and decided to tap with his fingertips under Mary's eyes (an end point of the *stomach meridian*). To his astonishment she announced immediately that her phobia was gone and she raced down to Callahan's swimming pool and began to throw water in her face. No fear. No headaches. It all went away –

including the nightmares – and has never returned. She is totally free of her water phobia.

Dr. Callahan tried tapping on a wide variety of mental problems: fear of heights, depression, fear for people, anxieties, panic disorders, worries, nightmares, post traumatic stress disorder, and other negative emotion, and found that many of his clients experienced great relief from their problems (in just minutes) – sometimes even for good.

Gary Craig, a Stanford engineer, opened this discovery up to a wider public and wrote a manual that is available on the Internet. In it he writes that "The true cause of negative emotions, it turns out, is not where everyone thinks it is. It is not where psychologists have been looking. That is why they haven't found it. They have been looking at the wrong place. *The cause of all negative emotions is found where disruptions take place in the body's energy system.*"

By tapping with the finger tips, energy is applied to places of the body that are "energy-sensitive", especially the endpoints of "meridians" (pathways of flowing energy). The effect of the tapping is that something happens in the nervous system – or better, in the energy system. Past bad experiences are being stripped of their negative emotional overload. You could say that, after doing the tapping, the experience does not hurt anymore, emotionally.

Gary's website is stocked with case-histories that one can freely browse through, and it is exciting to read the beautiful miracles that have happened through this simple method.

A VA hospital asked Gary to come and share his stuff with the vets. Imagine a Vietnam veteran who has not been able to live a normal life ever since his war experiences in the jungle caused him to have horrible nightmares and hallucinations. Therapists had worked with him for years and years, with hardly any success. Gary spent thirty minutes with one of them, after which the vet told him that, although the remembrance of the event is still there, the emotions that plagued him for so long have disappeared. The fear is gone. The anxiety is gone. The nightmares and hallucinations did not return.

Isn't that great stuff? Isn't that exciting! Imagine having a little tool with you that you can use at any time to take the sting out of every rotten experience or bad memory that you ever had in your life! It is exactly what we need: a fast and simple way to take the emotional overload away from our past experiences, so that they cannot any longer cause us to fear, worry, or live in anxiety or depression. Remember that it was these **negative emotions** that activate our stomach to produce acid twenty-four hours per day. They lower our pH, resulting in acidosis, which eventually can set the stage for the development of cancer.

> *"EFT is the single most effective tool I've learned in 40 years of being a therapist."*
> -- Dr. Steel, MD

Gary Craig gave a name to his "madness": Emotional Freedom Technique, or EFT. He graciously allowed part of his manual to be included in this book. To keep the volume of it to a minimum I will not go into all the why's, how's or what's. I will, instead, give you the most important parts of his tool box, the ones you can use *right now*.

EFT can be done by practically anyone, and you do not necessarily need the help of a professional, unless you are dealing with severe mental problems. So let's take a closer look at this method and see how you can apply it to your particular problem.

Although the full basic recipe consists of three parts, I will only introduce you to the first two, since most of the results are established when doing only these and I promised to keep it simple. Here they are:

1. The Setup
2. The Sequence

Part 1: The Setup. Imagine having to fire a rifle to hit a distant object. After loading it with the right caliber bullet there are certain things you have to do to hit the target. You have to set the scope for the right distance, then shoulder it, aim and pull the trigger. So it is with EFT. We need to do a couple of things to make sure we will hit the target of our problem bull's eye.

In the setup phase we set the scope and aim at the problem by saying a setup sentence and by tapping on a certain spot. The setup sentence consists of: the problem we're tapping for wrapped in an affirmation. Here are some examples of set-up sentences:

- *Even though I have **this constant fear of people**, I deeply and completely accept myself.*
- *Even though I **worry about my weight** so much, I deeply love and appreciate myself.*
- *Even though I have this **anger towards my father**, I completely accept and love myself.*
- *Even though I have these **anxiety attacks when I go shopping**, I deeply and completely accept myself.*

Why do I have to say: *"I deeply accept or love myself?"* you'll ask. Good question. The affirmation neutralizes a psychological phenomenon that is called "Psychological Reversal", which is like self sabotage. It is the reason why some diseases are chronic and respond very poorly to conventional treatments. It is also the reason why, for example, some people have such a difficult time losing weight. On the one hand they would really love to drop some weight, but on the other hand being overweight can help to cover other psychological issues. For example, someone who has been sexually abused in the past can use weight to literally cover up physical attraction.

When psychologically reversed somehow your energy does not flow the way it is supposed to go. It's like putting in the batteries of your flashlight the wrong way around; it won't work.

You do not feel when you have this psychological reversal. Only a few people are affected by this, even people with a very positive outlook on life. So, in order to be sure it won't hinder anyone we'll mention the affirmation in each sentence.

The second thing you'll have to do in the set-up is tapping with two or three of the middle fingers on the side of your other hand halfway between the base of the little finger and the top of the wrist. Gary calls it the karate chop point (KC). So while you say (aloud) the set-up sentence, at the same time you tap on the KC point (Left or right side makes no difference).

Again, the set-up looks like this: at least three times you speak out loud the set-up sentence while, at the same time, you tap on the KC point. It helps to put feeling and emphasis into the "I really love and appreciate myself..." part. When you speak out something, the ears will pick it up and feed it back to the brain. Emotions originate from a separate part of your brain. When you use emphasis in saying the set-up sentence, you'll involve this part of your brain in the set up even more.

Part 2: The Sequence. Now that we have zoomed in and aimed at the target, we can pull the trigger. Tapping is like shooting at the target, or better, at the problem we are now focused on.

The sequence is very simple in concept. It involves tapping on the end points of some of the major energy meridians in the body. To stay focused on your problem you want to speak it out, every time you move from one point to another. So if "angry at my father" is the problem, then just say "angry at my father" every time you change to a different point to tap on. This is what Gary calls the **Reminder Phrase**. (In the example set-up sentences on the previous page under Part 1, the reminder phrases are in bold.)

Before locating these tapping points, you need a few tips on how to carry out the tapping process.

Tapping tips. You can tap with either hand but it is usually more convenient to do so with your dominant hand (e.g. right hand if you are right handed). Tap with two or three fingertips. This covers a larger area than just tapping with one fingertip and allows you to cover the tapping points more easily. (If you have long fingernails, you may want to cut them or use the knuckles of your fingers instead)

Tap solidly but never so hard as to hurt or bruise yourself. Tap about seven to ten times on each of the tapping points. Most of the points exist on either side of the body. It doesn't matter which side you use, nor does it matter if you switch sides during the sequence. For example, you can tap under your right eye and, later in the sequence, tap under your left arm.

The tapping points. What follows are instructions on how to locate the end points of those meridians that we are going to tap on. Taken together and done in the order presented they form the sequence.

- At the beginning of the eyebrow, just above and to one side of the nose. This point is abbreviated **EB** for beginning of the **E**ye**B**row.

- On the bone bordering the outside corner of the eye. This point is called **SE** for **S**ide of the **E**ye.

- On the bone under the eye about 1 inch below your pupil. This is the **UE** point, for Under the Eye.

- On the small area between the bottom of your nose and the top of your upper lip. This point is abbreviated **UN** for Under the Nose.

- Midway between the point of your chin and the bottom of your lower lip. This point is **Ch** for **Chin.**

- The junction where the sternum (breastbone), collarbone and the first rib meet. To locate it, first place your forefinger on the U-shaped notch at the top of the breastbone (about where a man would knot his tie). From the bottom of the U, move your forefinger down toward the navel 1 inch and then go to the left (or right) one inch. This point is abbreviated **CB** for Collar Bone. It is a sensitive spot.

- On the side of the body and under the arm, at a point even with the nipple (for men) or in the middle of the bra strap (for women). It is about 4 inches below the armpit.
This point is abbreviated **UA** for Under the Arm.

Let's review:
KC = Karate Chop
EB = Beginning of the EyeBrow
SE = Side of the Eye
UE = Under the Eye

UN = Under the Nose
Ch = Chin
CB = Beginning of the Collar Bone
UA = Under the Arm

It should be a snap to memorize these eight points. A few trips through it and it should be yours forever.

The Reminder Phrase. Do not forget to speak out the reminder phrase. It is very important to stay focused on your problem when you do the tapping.

The basic recipe needs to be aimed at a specific problem. Otherwise, it will bounce around aimlessly with little or no effect. You aim the basic recipe, by applying it while "tuned in" to the problem from which you want relief. This tells your system which problem needs to be the receiver.

Remember the discovery statement which states,

> "The cause of all negative emotions is a disruption in the body's energy system."

Negative emotions come about because you are tuned in to certain thoughts or circumstances which cause your energy system to disrupt. Otherwise, you function normally. A fear of heights is not present, for example, while you're reading the comic section of the Sunday newspaper (and therefore you're not tuned in to the problem).

Tuning in to a problem can be done by simply thinking about it. Thinking about the problem will bring about the energy disruptions involved, which then and only then can be balanced by applying the basic recipe. That's why you need to make a reminder phrase that you can repeat continually while you are performing The Basic Recipe. The reminder phrase is simply a word or short phrase that describes the problem and that you repeat out loud each time you tap one of the points in the sequence. In this way you continually "remind" your system about the problem you are working on. Often adjustments are needed.

Let's say you are using the basic recipe for some problem (fear, headache, anger, etc.). Sometimes the problem will simply vanish after just one round while at other times one round provides only partial relief. When only partial relief is obtained, you will need to do one or more additional rounds. Those subsequent rounds need to be adjusted slightly for best results.

Or you have already made some headway but have become stopped partway toward complete relief because psychological reversal enters in a manner that keeps you from getting any better. Since the subconscious mind tends to be very literal, subsequent rounds of the basic recipe need to address the fact that you are working on the remaining problem. Accordingly, the affirmation contained within the setup needs to be adjusted as does the reminder phrase.

Here's the adjusted format for the setup affirmation: "Even though I *still* have *some* of this_____, I deeply and completely accept myself." Please note that the emphasized words change the thrust of the affirmation toward the remainder of the problem. It should be easy to make this adjustment and, after a little experience, you will fall into it quite naturally.

The reminder phrase is also easily adjusted. Just put the word *remaining* before the previously used phrase. Here, as examples, are adjusted versions of the previous reminder phrases:

... remaining fear of people,
... remaining worry about my weight,
... remaining anger towards my father.

Practice a couple of times and you'll see that you can master this protocol in no time.

While you tune into a problem or hang-up it will help you to score the measure of emotional or physical disturbance on a scale of zero to ten. Just ask yourself: how badly do I feel about this, or what is my pain level right now? Do it before and after a few rounds of tapping and see if you make progress.

On the EFT website, *www.emofree.com*, you can read fabulous case histories of people who were helped by EFT. EFT, as a way of re-setting or re-tuning one's energy system is a great tool.

A warning is in place though: many of the people that practice EFT as professional counselors often are also practitioners of techniques that this author does not endorse, like hypnosis. I advise you to stay far away from any technique or method that tries to influence or mess with your spirit. As a Christian I am strongly opposed to any spiritual counseling that is not based in a personal relationship with Jeshua, the Messiah.

Appendix B

Therapeutic use of Vitamin C

Linus Pauling, two-time Nobel prize winner, wrote in his book *How to Live Longer and Feel Better*: ["It has been recognized for many years that patients with cancer have a decreased level of Vitamin C in the blood ..." And: "The low level of vitamin C in the blood should, of course, be rectified for all cancer patients by a high intake of the vitamin C.'"]

Vitamin C (Ascorbic acid) is an excellent immune system booster. There is an avalanche of research material available dealing with the therapeutic use of vitamin C in the fight against cancer. Although the FDA's Recommended Daily Allowance (RDA) for vitamin C is approximately 1000 mg. per day, most research sources will advice amounts of 3000 mg to 10,000 mg per day, which may seem to be very much; however the research results are indicating that these "high" amounts establish far greater results than 1000 mg. per day.

Consider the following. Most mammals make vitamin C in their livers. We humans, as well as some type of ape, a bat and the guinea pig, have lost the ability to make our own vitamin C. Researchers have calculated that, compared to the daily intake of vitamin C by mammals, the equivalent amount of vitamin C per body weight for people is approximately 2000 - 4000 milligrams under conditions of little to no stress, but up to 15,000 milligrams under stressful conditions.[Irwin Stone; *The Healing Factor*] Being of the human race and living in the extremely stressful conditions of our Western culture, we should be taking a daily amount of 15,000 milligrams (or fifteen grams) of vitamin C.

The human liver has somehow been genetically disabled to produce ascorbic acid (vitamin C). So, the only way for us to get that amount per day is to eat a small truckload of green leafy vegetables, washed away with gallons of fresh orange juice. Now apes, bats and guinea pigs are known for their high intake of vitamin C through their diet. We Americans are known for not eating any vegetables!

The bottom line is this: in order to stay away from suffering from a chronic (lifelong) case of scurvy, we may have to supplement daily with five to ten grams of vitamin C! Drinking orange juice (fifty mg per glass) and even becoming a vegetarian is not going to cut it. That advice was for healthy people. For people who suffer from disease, like cancer, a more therapeutic approach will be helpful:

15,000 milligrams, divided over twenty-four hours, is a normal and healthy amount (625 mg per hour). Taking a 500 mg tablet of vitamin C every half hour during a day of 15 hours would probably be the best compromise. Linus Pauling writes about **"bowel tolerance"** as an indication of how much vitamin C one can handle. When you start to get loose bowels you know that you have taken too much of it. Pauling advises (cancer) patients who use vitamin C in therapeutic amounts, to stay just under this effect of loose bowels. Gradually build up your vitamin C dose until the point where you get loose bowels, then take a little less and stay there.

The consumption of vitamin C is also very important when going through (cancer) surgery. Research has shown that on the days after surgery, the amount of vitamin C in the blood serum drops to an almost negligible level. It indicates the vital function of vitamin C in the fabrication of new tissue. Before you go for surgery, load up on vitamin C!

Smokers "burn" away forty mg. of vitamin C per cigarette. On top of that they damage the lining of their lungs with the free radicals in the smoke, which increases the need for vitamin C.

When you go for X-rays or radiation treatment, the tissues that are targeted receive a high dose of free-radicals that, as a side effect, can damage the healthy parts of your body. Vitamin C acts as a vital defender by neutralizing much of these free-radicals.

You have read that as a cancer patient it is critical that you receive direct sunlight on your skin. Vitamin C taken before and after your time in the sun will give you some protection so you will not burn as easily. Living in Florida close to the beaches, I have found out many times that vitamin C protects against sunburn.

Vitamin C is not a cause of kidney stones, as some medical people try to make you believe; as a matter of fact it helps to prevent stones from forming in your kidneys. The only known side effect of taking too much vitamin C is: loose bowels, which can be a blessing when you're constipated.

A high dose of vitamin C has also been shown to be effective as a transporter of oxygen in combination with vitamin E. Vitamin C transports oxygen in the *water-based* cell bodies and vitamin E in the *oil-based* membranes. Both work together as partners, inhibiting cancer by enhancing oxygen uptake by tumor tissue.

According to William Campbell Douglass II, MD, new research shows that high doses of intravenous (IV) vitamin C can fight cancer, an effect first suggested back in the 1970s. According to the study, published in an issue of [The Proceedings of the National Academy of Sciences], intravenous vitamin C led to the formation of hydrogen peroxide in the blood. This process caused the destruction of many cancer cells, while leaving healthy cells undisturbed. Hydrogen peroxide is a very potent molecule with an extra oxygen atom bound to it (H_2O_2), which can be released to fight off disease.

It will not be easy, but try to find a doctor who is willing and able to treat you in this way. A tiny needle will be inserted into a blood vessel of your arm; the doctor will hook up a small tube between the needle and a bag with a vitamin C solution. Just sit down and relax; in a few hours the solution will drip into your bloodstream to enrich it with a very healthy cancer fighter.

Using vitamin C is *not* just making "expensive urine," as some people say. They do not understand that the only way to increase the concentration of vitamin C in your tissues is by flooding your bloodstream with it. And since blood also circulates through the kidneys, these filters will strain away some of the vitamin C, which you'll find in your yellow-colored urine. At the same time, the tissues everywhere else in your body will also suck up the necessary vitamin C. Yellow urine is OK. If it wouldn't be yellow it wouldn't be safe to eat any snow anywhere at all!

There is enough sound scientific evidence to conclude that the intake of high amounts of vitamin C prevents cancer, stunts tumor growth, and plays a role in affecting programmed cell death of tumor cells.

Appendix C

Horror Stories

Of course this little book is not complete in showing you all the different alternative approaches to cancer control. Every year more discoveries are being made by the zealous work of scientists who have dedicated their life and work to their suffering neighbors.

Dr. Wilburn Ferguson   is the man whose life inspired the movie: *'Medicine man,'* starring Sean Connery. Of course the story in the movie was changed to a more politically correct fable. Here is the real story:

Dr. Ferguson, through many adventurous trials, engaged in a relationship with a head-hunter medicine-man in the South American jungle by saving his child from disease. Grateful for his son's healing the head-hunter "doctor" gave Ferguson a bottle of herbal fluid that had been used for thousands of years in the process of shrinking enemy heads.

After testing it on some of his patients, Ferguson discovered that this herbal brew was a very potent and safe anti-cancer formula. After trying it out on several patients and curing most of them from cancer and ulcers, he took a sample of it to different drug companies in the U.S.A., to have it researched. They too established incredible results with the formula, but Ferguson ended up being ridiculed by the leaders of modern medicine. They refused to do further research because, as they told him: it is simply too good and it will ruin our cancer business. Ferguson, frustrated, went back to his patients in the jungle!

Royal Raymond Rife built a microscope that was more powerful than anyone had built before. He discovered life forms no one had ever seen before and found a cure for cancer in 1934. When Rife, wanting his discoveries to benefit all of mankind, refused to sell his protocol and equipment to the authorities of the American Medical Association, his research laboratory was destroyed and his equipment broken to pieces and stolen. Cancer could have been eradicated in America before the second World War!

Gaston Naessens, a sixty-nine-year-old French microbiologist, discovered a cancer treatment, he calls his immune-system therapy: 714X. His findings run parallel to Rife's discovery of a cancer virus. When Naessens' unorthodox treatment methods began yielding dramatic successes in his native France, French medical authorities closed his lab, confiscated his equipment, and heavily fined him for practicing medicine without a license. After going to Canada he set up a small laboratory outside Montreal, but was taken to court. After a long trial, in which numerous testimonies were offered by patients and physicians using his approach, he was finally acquitted. Now, a handful of doctors are struggling to make Naessens' controversial treatments readily available.

Dr. Patrick Flannagan made the truly revolutionary discovery of charging the hydrogen molecule with an extra electron (microhydrin), after years and years of agonizing research.

Dr. Hulda Clark recently was locked up in jail for several days, being over seventy years old. She too has found a cure for cancer, with a caseload of recovered patients to prove it. The medical 'establishment' is after her too and tries to make her cancer research impossible.

Dr. Ryke Geerd Hamer is locked up in a French jail as this is written, accused of practicing medicine without a license. His approach to cancer treatment is too successful, so the medical establishment pulled away his license and arrested him when he courageously continued treating cancer patients.

The "Wellness Directory of Minnesota" graciously allowed me to print their article about Dr. Sam Chachoua, M.B.B.S. (the Australian version of M.D.) and his unbelievable struggle with the powers that be after he found a vaccine for cancer.

I'll just sit back now and let them tell you the story:

In the Beginning....
A young boy in Australia watched his father die slowly from multiple myeloma, a terrible form of cancer that does not respond to

chemotherapy or radiation. With every new medicine hope grew and grew until it just ran out as his father got sicker and sicker. This bright young teen felt driven by his father's suffering. The news was filled with breakthroughs in cancer, but still his father lay dying a horribly painful death as his bones began to crush under the weight of his body.

Sam Chachoua felt his calling. He would be a doctor, despite the limitations of modern medicine he had witnessed in those painful years. However, because of those same limitations, Sam decided early on that the secret lay elsewhere, way beyond the toxic chemicals and radiation that, to him, either killed or cured, and sometimes left the patient worse off than the disease itself.

He began to question the way in which modern medicine looked at cancer. He began to investigate the phenomenon of "spontaneous remission", why in some people the cancer just went away and why some organs seem to fight off cancers better than others do. He was driven not by fame and fortune, but by the memory of his father. He would find a way to cure cancer and end suffering.

At the age of eighteen, Sam Chachoua (pronounced Cha-choo -wa) presented an original paper on cancer before the Clinical Oncology Society of Australia. He was the youngest presenter ever. He graduated from medical school with honors and as his research into curing cancer took off, he also developed some very effective therapies against a host of ailments using non-toxic medicines. Dr. Chachoua believed firmly in the first law of medicine: Do no harm. It made no sense to him to stress the body or disrupt the immune system in an attempt to cure a disorder. This thinking remained the foundation of his cancer research.

While focusing on those factors that trigger spontaneous remission, Dr. Chachoua developed sera (the plural of serum), extracts, and vaccines. He recognized that in cancer, as well as in AIDS, the immune system has trouble recognizing diseased tissue. Cancer has a real bad habit of hiding from the immune system. In metastases, cancer cells bond with fibrin (the clotting agent in the blood) and travels throughout the body unrecognized by the immune system. Dr. Chachoua also studied the immune response; the various triggers in the body once it spots an invader like a cold or flu virus. He theorized that if he could "tag" a cancer cell with a cold or flu virus, the cancer would no longer be able to hide from the immune system, and would light up like a Hollywood movie premiere.

Chachoua's sera consisted of concentrated genetic materials that could tag cancer cells (or cells infected with AIDS, damaged heart cells, and even damaged brain cells in Alzheimer's patients). With healthy cells, foreign genetic materials will be attacked and destroyed if they attempt to infiltrate. However, diseased cells do not have this response. Additionally, Dr. Chachoua studied autoimmune diseases (such as lupus and rheumatoid arthritis) realizing that this response held therapeutic potential, as patients suffering from these diseases could provide him with cultures that could save the lives of others. Patients with lupus lack enzymes to digest invaders, so the immune system compensates with a very unique response that enters cells for correction or defense.

Dr. Chachoua borrowed his theories from the wisdom of the body itself. Today, his Induced Remission Therapy (IRT) has no equal in the annals of medicine. The effectiveness of his sera and vaccines is unequaled and for those who are terrified at the prospects of an AIDS vaccine passing on the AIDS virus, Dr. Chachoua's vaccines consist of healthy cells, not diseased cells. There is no cancer in his cancer vaccine; there is no HIV, no virus, dead or alive, in his AIDS vaccine.

Dr. Chachoua's sera and vaccines have been tested. They've proven to be 99% effective. Nothing in the history of medicine has proven to be 99% effective against cancers and AIDS, which begs the question, "Why haven't we heard of Dr. Chachoua?"

Those of us who have heard of Dr. Chachoua in the past probably didn't hear of him in a good light. Quackwatch, a web site dedicated to promoting the hard lined AMA/Pharmaceutical Company interests, calls Chachoua a confirmed quack and crybaby suing everyone for his failures. The news media has, on numerous occasions, called him a quack and a charlatan, at times resorting to claims that he's never had any medical training.

That is, up until August, 2000, when NBC news headlined this story: THE MOST

EFFECTIVE THERAPY AGAINST CANCER
AND AIDS IN HISTORY.

What caused this change? Very simply, Dr.
Chachoua sued his detractors in court and won
a 10 million dollar settlement. When you win,
even NBC, the network that has lied to us
about vitamins and minerals, about the
dangers of organic foods, about the efficacy of
alternative practices, even they had to finally
tell us the truth, after he took his detractors to
court and won.

Modern Medicine:
Welcome to the obstacle course!

Dr. Chachoua developed his theories, his sera,
and his vaccines on his own. Not affiliated with
a large university or a pharmaceutical company,
he's not found an easy path. His papers went
unpublished. His work went ignored. To prove
his theories, he's traveled the world over giving
lectures, curing patients with cancer, heart
disease, AIDS, and Alzheimer's. He offered
anyone willing to prove or disprove his theories
an unprecedented half a million dollars. It
looked like no one would take up his offer until
he connected up with Cedars-Sinai Medical
Center. They designed a program to test IRT, but
Chachoua would have to turn over all his
research and all his sera; holding back nothing.
Chachoua, thinking they were seriously
interested, did just this. Early results were
spectacular as Cedars reported a 99% cure and

claimed to have discovered in Chachoua's IRT an "exciting new world of therapeutic opportunity!"

Then Dr. Chachoua's world began to systematically fall apart. Some people, former acquaintances and associates of Chachoua's and supporters who he had cured using his IRT, opened a clinic in Mexico claiming to be affiliated with the good doctor. They showed videos of his speaking engagements and sold vials of water at exorbitant prices to people seeking cures. People died, fingers pointed, the scandal grew. Chachoua quickly had the clinics closed, but then they'd open under another name. He even went to Mexico to personally put a stop to these charlatans when he was arrested. He could not prove he was a real medical doctor (who carries their diploma with them) and the Mexican authorities had been bribed by the charlatans to lock him away.

This was just the excuse Cedars-Sinai Medical Center needed. They denied ever having any relationship with him, issued press releases stating this, and denied ever testing his sera and vaccines.

Instead of giving Dr. Chachoua credit for his research, one of the principle investigators who had tested Chachoua's vaccines, wrote and published a paper on the possibilities of curing cancer and AIDS with sera from people with autoimmune disease.

We could go on, telling you how much grief Dr. Chachoua had to endure. Let's face it, Chachoua's association with Cedars-Sinai Medical Center began in 1996. The trial ended in

August of 2000. That's four full years of abuse, and at the trial one witness even exclaimed that Cedars had committed "premeditated manslaughter" because of the number of lives lost to AIDS alone during this 4 year struggle.

Chachoua endured hell during this time from physical attacks to threats on his life and the entire medical profession all over him like fleas on a Tennessee hound dog. The 10 million dollar verdict is nothing compared to the loss of life during this period, or the loss of dignity of this human being whose only desire was to cure the sick. But it was enough to get NBC to finally tell the truth about an alternative cure for cancer.

The trial was exciting, though. Every time Cedars made a claim, a letter was brought out to prove them to be liars. We never tested it: poof, a letter showing the results. They never tested toxicity: poof, a letter showing they could not explain how they were so nontoxic and yet they powerfully inhibited the HIV virus.

The final blow came when a person suffering from AIDS was called to testify. Cedars never returned Dr. Chachoua's sera. The good doctor was bankrupt. He could not possibly make more of his vaccines, but he did have one dose of his most powerful vaccine left; something he'd held back from Cedars. This last remaining dose just might have achieved more for humanity than any other medicine in history.

Michael arrived to testify. He'd been taking conventional protease inhibitors, the drug cocktail promoted by Cedars for years as everything but the cure. His T-cell count had deteriorated to 124 as the virus took hold of him. However, when asked how he felt, he responded "Exceptionally well." When asked why he felt well, he told the jury that he'd had a dose of Dr. Chachoua's vaccine the previous day and that his immune function had doubled (T-cells rising to over 200). In other words, he had gone from full-blown AIDS to remission in one day.

When asked by Chachoua's attorney, "And how do you know that your immune system doubled?" he responded that he'd had several blood tests taken. Where? "Cedars-Sinai Medical Center," replied Michael.

The verdict was unanimous.

Induced Remission Therapy

Ten million bucks is nothing in a world of medicine controlled by a multi-billion dollar cartel we know as the Pharmaceutical industry.

We focused on AIDS above in our description of the trial, but Chachoua's own research has shown his sera to be just as effective on cancer, heart disease (growing back diseased tissues modern medicine says is impossible to re-grow), and Alzheimer's (growing back brain cells).

Now that the truth is out, you can expect more and more news releases on "genetic" cures for cancer to be in the headlines. The race is on. Everyone wants to beat Dr. Chachoua to the punch. The big players, cancer institutes, pharmaceutical industries, major university medical schools all want to beat Dr. Chachoua at the game of curing cancer. No more wasted money. For years every donation to some cancer organization put some researcher's kid, some doctor's kid, some association president's kid through college while cancer patients suffered and died at the same rates since WWII. We've been lied to, beaten up, and buried. But now, with a cancer cure recognized by a jury of twelve and announced by NBC news, the cure will have to come.

Only one hurdle stands in front of Dr. Chachoua: the FDA. Now, if we'd all written our representatives in Congress and in the Senate, this step might not be necessary. The FDA must approve a drug based upon effectiveness. Yes, they check safety, but to be approved it has to work, and that costs money and takes time. To prove it is safe is relatively easy and cheap.

Had we all written our representatives asking them to pass the Health Freedom act, which would allow us to use any medicine (even unproven) as long as it has proven itself to be safe, we'd all have access to Induced Remission Therapy. But we don't. Yet.

Update on Dr. Chachoua, September 2001

The judge reversed himself on a technicality and awarded Dr. Chachoua his original investment of eleven thousand dollars. This means that Dr. Chachoua is bankrupt. After battling the system for ten years, Dr. Chachoua wins the battle but loses the war. He is so broke he cannot even purchase the organisms he needs to create his cures.

Dr. Chachoua's organization came to us recently asking for help. They discovered this article and were very impressed at our reporting. They had hoped we could help them get a study going here in America. I am doing my damndest, making phone calls, writing letters, etc., but we here at the Wellness Directory of Minnesota are mere volunteers and we have little pull in the world of medicine.

Dr. Chachoua wants to do a study on heart disease or AIDS. He refuses to touch cancer anymore because the Cancer Industry is just too powerful. Isn't that wonderful. The Cancer Industry, after searching for a cure for some 40 years spending/earning some gazillion dollars for their struggle, have finally had their first major victory: they have suppressed a cancer cure that would have put them out of business. They've finally guaranteed the deaths of hundreds of thousands of individuals. They can do all this, and still show a profit. Ahhh, ya gotta love em.

Dr. Chachoua will do anything to get a study going. I am currently in contact with a few universities, and we'll see what they have to offer. His organization has contacted hundreds of AIDS organizations, but since they are funded by our government, no one wants to help him with a study, even though he proved in a court of law that he can cure AIDS. Our government just doesn't want to cure AIDS yet; there are just too many undesirables out there with the bug.

What I see happening is Dr. Chachoua will go to Africa or Asia where they do want to cure AIDS because it is a rampant epidemic. Or, Dr. Chachoua will die and his cures will die with him. Because he is working at a genetic level, here is what his therapies can do:

- Reverse AIDS for a period of six months to a year.
- Reverse cardiac myopathy (dead tissue is replaced with healthy tissue) and scar tissue in the heart.
- Reverse atherosclerosis without surgery.
- Repair a heart valve without surgery.
- Reverse nearly all forms of cancer (especially the deadliest ones).

If anyone out there has any idea where Dr. Chachoua can get a study done, please contact us at 763-689-9355.

Perhaps you know a rich person who is dying of one of the above maladies? This is what it's going to take. It is going to take money. Hell, look how much we've spent already and gotten what in return? The Poison of the Month Club. Buy 12 poisons for a penny each and just one more poison at regular rates, and if it works, fine, if it doesn't, too bad.

Update on Dr. Chachoua
November 2001

Dr. Sam has been taking a beating by our judicial system. He's out of money and cannot afford to fight back. So, he's losing. We all know in America that justice goes to whoever can afford it. So with his health failing, the courts reversing practically everything so that they've left the door open so his detractors may now sue him, and his detractors slandering his name all over the country, Dr. Sam is not finding many supporters. Ever web sites that once spoke highly of him are suddenly silent. Most have disappeared.

The good new is this: because of you and us together, we have found three (possibly) four locations that might be able to help Dr. Sam test his therapy. He will probably be leaving America. Africa sure can use him, seeing how people are dying by the thousands with AIDS.

Watch the News Program that tells all about the Cedars-Sinai Medical Center Lawsuit
When you can go on the internet enter the following:
http://www.mnwelldir.org/docs/Newsletters/images/CancerCure(350k)[1].mov to see a video with the news program. It's very big (8MB) and the sound is bad in spots, but it's the only REAL proof we have that our story is true.

Dr. Chachoua Update
June 2005

Dr. San Chachoua is in good health and is away researching another theory he's come up with. However, his therapies for HIV/AIDS, Heart Disease, and Cancer are now available. All you need is a physician willing to administer it.

The price is $10,000.00 per therapy. Each therapy is administered in seven injections over a 15 day period. People with cardiovascular disease report that they begin to feel better within minutes of the first injections.

If you want to discuss this, ask questions, or order the therapy, contact Gilbert at phbal@msn.com.

Thank you "Wellness Directory of Minnesota." It is a powerful testimony of the sick reality in cancer research land.

The Wellness Directory of Minnesota website is: *www.mnwelldir.org* or email: *info@mnwelldir.org.*

Recommended Reading

Alive and Well, one doctor's experience with nutrition *(laetrile)* in the treatment of cancer patients. Philip E. Binzel Jr., M.D. The heroic fight of a family doctor who takes on the medical establishment and helps cure his patients of cancer.

Laetrile Case Histories, sixty-two case histories proving that laetrile (vitamin B_{17}) works in the control of cancer. By John A. Richardson, M.D. and Patricia Irving Griffin, R.N., B.S.

World Without Cancer, the story of vitamin B_{17}, by G. Edward Griffin. An in-depth history of vitamin B_{17}. Description of how it works and what cancer is. The second part of the book is all about the politics behind cancer therapy. A must if you want to understand how things could go so wrong in America. Reads like a detective novel. Edward Griffin's website: www.realityzone.com.

The Cure for All Diseases, The Cure for All Cancers, and *The Cure for All Advanced Cancers.* Hulda Regehr Clark, Ph.D., N.D. Read the protocols of her cancer cures. Read the many testimonies. Fascinating stuff! Website about Dr. Clark's books:

www.drclark.net or about her products: www.drclark.com.

The Cancer Answer. Albert E. Carter. About the importance of a proper functioning immune system in relation to cancer.

The Cancer Cure that Worked. Barry Lynes writes about fifty years of suppression of a cancer-cure that worked. The history of Royal R. Rife, a genius researcher and inventor, and about the American Medical Society's dirty politics.

Why Christians Get Sick. Dr. George H. Malkmus survived colon cancer and writes about the "Genesis-diet". Important eye-openers. Dr. Malkmus's website: www.hacres.com.

Your Body's Many Cries for Water. F. Batmanghelidj, M.D. Why dehydration is the cause of many diseases. Fascinating testimonies. Dr. Batmanghelidj's website: www.watercure.com.

Flax Oil as a True Aid against Arthritis, Heart Infarction, Cancer and Other Diseases. Dr. Johanna Budwig. This remarkable lady has brought about a scientific revolution about the relationship between cancer research and fat metabolism.

Understanding Fats and Oils: Your Guide to Healing with Essential Fatty Acids Michael T. Murray, N.D. and Jade Beutler, R.R.T., R.C.P.

The Calcium Factor and *Death By Diet,* Robert R. Barefoot and Carl J. Reich, M.D. Essential knowledge about the acid - alkaline balance in relation to cancer. Bob Barefoot's website: www.cureamerica.net.

How to Live Longer and Feel Better. Linus Pauling, two-time Nobel Prize winner writes about the need for vitamins and minerals. A must-read classic!

What Your Doctor May Not Tell You About Menopause. John R. Lee, M.D. A life-saving book about the dangers of hormone replacement therapies and the healthy alternatives. Explains everything. For women and for men.

Alkalize or Die. Dr. Theodore A. Baroody, N.D.,D.C.,Ph.D. Nutrition, C.N.C. Lots of information about the alkaline-acid balance, with menu planning and recipes.

Oxygen, Dr. Kurt Donsbach, D.C., N.D., Ph. D. All about simple Oxygen therapies that you can do by yourself.

O2Xygen Therapies: A New Way of Approaching Disease, and *Flood Your Body with Oxygen,* by Ed McCabe. A must-read, all about oxygen therapies. Ed's website: www.oxygenhealth.com.

The Healing Factor, Vitamin C's important role in your body's fight against disease. By Irwin Stone.

The Healing Field, restoring the positive energy of health. By Dr. M.T. Morter, Jr.

Prescription For Disaster, a DVD documentary about the symbiotic relationship between the FDA, lobbyists, law-makers, medical schools and researchers and the impact it has on you, the consumer of healthcare. Written, produced and directed by Gary Null, PhD.

The Hidden Messages In Water, by Masaru Emoto. A wonderful book about the influence of speech and thoughts on the shape of water crystals.

When Healing Becomes A Crime, the amazing story of the Hoxsey Cancer Clinics and the return of alternative therapies. By Kenny Ausubel.

Sick and tired? About how to reclaim your inner terrain, your milieu. Robert O Young, Ph.D., D.Sc. with Shelley Redford Young, L.M.T.

The Bible, a rich source of healthy dietary guidelines, stress- and anger-management, relationship restoration and healthy community living. Teaching on prayer and meditation and a road map on how to get back in touch with the Creator. The book you should read when everything else has failed.

Interesting Health
Websites

---

www.vitamincfoundation.org - all about vitamin C.

www.cforyourself.com - more about vitamin C.

www.lef.com - Life Extention Foundation.

www.karlloren.com - general health, chelation.

www.4.dr-rath-foundation.org - general health.

www.thewolfeclinic.com - alternative healthcare.

www.cancure.org - all about cancer treatments.

www.curezone.com - more about cancer treatments.

www.mercola.com - general health. One of the largest balanced websites on health. Highly recommended.

www.doctoryourself.com - general health.

www.morter.com - acid/alkaline, health alternatives.

www.emofree.com - Emotional Freedom Technique.

www.mnwelldir.org - a wellness directory.

www.oxygenhealth.com - Ed McCabe's website.

www.learninggnm.com – Dr. R.G. Hamer's ideas explained.

Disclaimer

As you undoubtedly will know, The Food and Drug Administration (FDA) does not allow treatments to be claimed as cures without their stamp of approval. This approval can only be obtained after very extensive and expensive scientific tests and studies for which many independent researchers simply do not have the funds. However, even after all these tests and studies have been done, history has shown that many of the drugs that **were** approved by the FDA, years later appeared to be extremely dangerous for public use. Examples are Baycol, Vioxx and Prozac, which in recent years have caused suffering and death of a multitude of people.

So we all need to ask ourselves: who is kidding whom!

In October 2005 the cherry industry was warned by the FDA to stop publicizing scientific data about the health benefits of cherry products. Why? Well, when you disseminate health information about a product, that product becomes a drug! An *unapproved* drug, that is. And claims about drugs can only be made by the FDA and by doctors. So cherry producers who claim health benefits are practicing medicine without a license and can be thrown in jail. Yes, read it again and scratch your head. Now, you'll understand why I write a disclaimer!

The statements in this book have not been evaluated by the Food and Drug Administration. The author of this book is *not* a medical doctor and cannot, does not want and does not mean to prescribe any treatment, medication or supplement. You are advised to consult an open minded health care professional before beginning any new dietary supplement program. In view of the possibility of human error, the author does not warrant that the information contained in this book is in every respect accurate or complete and he is not responsible, nor liable for any errors or omissions that may be found in this book, or for the results obtained from the use of such information. This book simply is a report about doctors who have found ways to successfully fight cancer, according to their own claims in literature.

I just report their findings. You decide!

After writing 'Away with Cancer' I studied further about Dr. R.G. Hamer's approach to cancer and, by reading his material, a whole new way of looking at health and healing opened up to me. With a 90% cure rate of cancer, this doctor simply blows many theories and practices out of the water. I also experienced in my own practicing of physical therapy that this doctor is the real deal.

I found, however, no non-medical books that would explain Dr. Hamer's theories to a wider and less informed public.

At the same time, breast cancer is till rampant; so much so that women chose to amputate their breasts to try to stay clear of breast cancer.

What a horrible situation!

I wrote "The Cause and Cure of Breast Cancer" to make women understand Dr. Hamer's approach to cancer and to give them the tools and weapons to make their fight a fair one.

I realize the pretense of writing the <u>cause</u> and <u>cure</u> of cancer into the title of the book, but I sincerely believe that Dr. Hamer has found both.

Any woman will need this book, not just to educate herself about the cause and the cure of breast cancer, but also to help, educate and support their friends and loved ones.

Be a rich blessing to your community!

You wanted to know...

THE CAUSE &
CURE OF
BREAST CANCER

Now... go win this fight!

DICK SCHUYT

BACHELORS DEGREE IN PHYSICAL EDUCATION AND PHYSICAL THERAPY

Contact

If the information in this book has helped
you get well, please let me know your story.

You can contact me by email:

AWAYWITHCANCER@AOL.COM

Or write me at the following address:

**P.O. BOX 144,
ROCKY FACE, GEORGIA, 30740**

For bulk-orders of
"the Cause and Cure of Breast Cancer"
or "Away with Cancer",
write or email me.

www.ingramcontent.com/pod-product-compliance
Lightning Source LLC
Chambersburg PA
CBHW051853170526
45168CB00001B/96